"Bounce Back Better: Your Trauma Healing Guide"

"9 Steps to Overcome Challenges, Heal Emotional Wounds, and Embrace Inner Strength: A Practical Guide"

Emotion Tutor

© Copyright 2023 – All rights reserved.

The content contained within this book may not be reproduced, duplicated, or transmitted without direct written permission from the author or the publisher. Under no circumstances will any blame or legal responsibility be held against the publisher, or author, for any damages, reparation, or monetary loss due to the information contained within this book. Either directly or indirectly.

Legal Notice:
This book is copyright protected. This book is only for personal use. You cannot amend, distribute, sell, use, quote, or paraphrase any part, or the content within this book, without the consent of the author or publisher.

Disclaimer Notice:
Please note the information contained within this document is for educational and entertainment purposes only. All effort has been executed to present accurate, up-to-date, and reliable complete information. No warranties of any kind are declared or implied. Readers acknowledge that the author is not rendering legal, financial, medical, or professional advice. The content within this book has been derived from various sources. Please consult a licensed professional before attempting any techniques outlined in this book. By reading this document, the reader agrees that under no circumstances is the author responsible for any direct or indirect losses incurred as a result of the use of the information contained within this document, including, but not limited to, errors, omissions, or inaccuracies.

Contents

1. Understanding Trauma — 1
2. Step 1 - Acceptance: Acknowledging Your Trauma — 8
3. Step 2 - Seek Support: Building Your Healing Network — 16
4. Step 3 - Self-Care: Prioritizing Your Well-being — 23
5. Step 4 - Therapy: Utilizing Professional Help — 30
6. Step 5 - Expression: Releasing Your Emotions — 37
7. Step 6 - Mindfulness: Cultivating Presence — 44
8. Step 7 - Resilience: Building Strength From Struggle — 53
9. Step 8 - Growth: Embracing Post-Traumatic Growth — 61
10. Step 9- Maintaining Progress and Preventing Relapse — 69
11. Moving Forward: Embracing a New Life After Trauma — 76

Chapter 1

Understanding Trauma

Life often presents us with challenging situations, but when these events are extraordinarily distressing, they may lead to trauma. Imagine yourself walking through a dense forest on a stormy night. Every rustle, every shadow, every sound feels threatening. That's what experiencing trauma can be like, an overwhelming and intense emotional response to a distressing event or series of events. Trauma shakes you to your core, causing emotional distress and even physical discomfort. These situations could range from a single event like a car accident or natural disaster to long-term situations like enduring abuse or neglect. The after-effects of such events can continue long after the incident itself, leaving deep emotional scars. You might find yourself reliving the traumatic event, struggling with persistent fear, or even feeling numb.

Yet, it's crucial to remember that experiencing trauma doesn't mean you're weak or broken. It's not about what's wrong with you, but rather what happened to you. Yes, trauma may change how you see the world, but it doesn't define you. You are more than the challenges you've faced. And the most empowering aspect? You have an incredible ability to heal and grow from your trauma. Emotional wounds, just like physical ones, need care, compassion, and time to heal. With these elements and the right resources, you can move forward, find strength in your journey, and even use your experiences to grow. So, let's embark on this healing journey together.

1.1: What is Trauma?

Trauma is a complex and deeply personal experience that can feel like an emotional earthquake, shaking up your life and leaving you feeling unsettled, hurt, and lost. It can come in many forms, such as the loss of a loved one, experiencing violence, surviving a natural disaster, or enduring long-term abuse or neglect. These experiences can feel overwhelming, causing intense emotional pain, fear, or even a sense of numbness. It's like your mind has been wounded. You may find yourself reliving the event in your mind, having nightmares or experiencing a constant sense of fear or dread. You may find it hard to trust others, to feel safe, or to believe that things will get better.

But it's important to remember that experiencing trauma doesn't mean you're weak or broken. It's a normal response to abnormal events. Trauma is not about what's wrong with you, but what happened to you. It's a sign that you've endured something difficult, but it doesn't define who you are. And here's the hopeful part: you have an incredible capacity to heal and grow from trauma. Just as a physical wound needs care and time to heal, emotional wounds also need compassion and patience. You can learn new ways to cope, to understand your emotions, and to build a life filled with meaning, purpose, and connection. Trauma may be a part of your story, but it doesn't have to be the end of it.

1.2: Types of Trauma

Trauma can occur in many forms and everyone experiences it differently. Here are some commonly recognized types of trauma:

a) Acute Trauma: This is often the result of a single, distressing event, such as a car accident, a natural disaster, or a violent attack. This sudden, intense trauma can cause both physical and emotional damage.

b) Chronic Trauma: This occurs when a person is exposed to multiple traumatic events over an extended period. This can include experiences like ongoing child abuse, domestic violence, or living in a war-torn region. The repeated nature of these events can make recovery more complex.

c) Complex Trauma: This type of trauma often happens in childhood, where an individual experiences multiple traumatic events, often invasive and interpersonal in nature. This might include prolonged abuse, neglect, or experiencing a traumatic event within a caregiving relationship, which disrupts a child's sense of safety and trust.

d) Secondary or Vicarious Trauma: This is experienced by those who are close to someone who has suffered trauma. For example, family members, friends, or therapists may absorb the traumatic experiences of those they're trying to help, leading to symptoms of trauma themselves.

e) Historical or Collective Trauma: These are traumas that affect entire communities, societies, or cultures. They can result from events like war, genocide, colonialism, or slavery. The effects of such traumas can be transmitted across generations.

f) Developmental Trauma: This type of trauma happens when a child's development is disrupted by early trauma, often within the context of a caregiver relationship. It can impact their ability to form healthy relationships, manage emotions, and develop a positive sense of self. Each type of trauma has its unique effects, but it's important to note that they can overlap.

1.3: How Trauma Affects You: Physically, Emotionally, and Psychologically

Trauma can leave a profound impact on a person, influencing not just their emotions and thoughts, but also their physical well-being. Here's how trauma can affect you on multiple levels:

Physically: When we experience a traumatic event, our bodies respond by activating the ""fight, flight, or freeze"" response. This is our body's survival mechanism, where adrenaline and cortisol, the stress hormones, are released. While this response can be life-saving in immediate danger, prolonged exposure to these stress hormones can have long-term effects on physical health. This can result in chronic health conditions such as heart disease, diabetes, or gastrointestinal problems. Moreover, trauma can disrupt sleep patterns, cause fatigue, headaches, and muscle tension. Some people may also experience changes in appetite and weight.

Emotionally: The emotional impact of trauma is complex and varied. Common reactions include feelings of fear, sadness, guilt, anger, and shame. A person may feel overwhelmed by these intense emotions and may struggle to manage them effectively. Some might become emotionally numb, feeling detached from their emotions as a protective measure. This emotional turmoil can lead to difficulties in forming and maintaining relationships, as trust and emotional intimacy may feel threatening to someone who has experienced trauma.

Psychologically: Trauma can lead to various psychological issues, the most common being Post-Traumatic Stress Disorder (PTSD). PTSD can involve intrusive memories or flashbacks of the event, avoidance of anything that reminds of the trauma, changes in thoughts and mood, and increased arousal symptoms like irritability and difficulty concentrating. Other potential psychological consequences include anxiety disorders, depression, and issues related to self-esteem and self-worth. It can also disrupt one's sense of safety, trust, and self-identity.

Trauma can also impact one's cognitive function, affecting memory and concentration. It can distort a person's beliefs about themselves and the world, often leading to a constant state of fear, helplessness, or feeling that the world is dangerous. It's crucial to note that not everyone who experiences trauma will have all these symptoms, and responses can change over time. Just as the impact of trauma is highly individual, so is the process of healing. The journey to recovery isn't linear, and it may involve setbacks, but with the right support and resources, individuals can navigate their path to healing and regain their sense of control and hope. Remember, experiencing trauma is not a sign of weakness. It's a testament to human resilience that we can endure such experiences and still continue to grow. The effects of trauma can be profound, but they don't define you. You are not alone in this journey, and help is available. In this guide, we'll explore strategies to help you heal from trauma, tap into your inner strength, and move towards a healthier, hopeful future.

1.4: Case Study: Examining personal stories and case studies can deepen our understanding of trauma and how it impacts individuals. Here are two real-life stories that illuminate the varied ways people can experience and respond to trauma.

Case Study 1: Jane

Jane is a 35-year-old woman who experienced acute trauma following a severe car accident. The accident left her with physical injuries and a newfound fear of driving. Physically, Jane suffered from chronic back pain, and the stress hormones released during the accident triggered digestive problems. Her once lively social life dwindled as she developed a fear of being in cars, even as a passenger.

Emotionally, Jane battled with recurring nightmares of the accident, leaving her feeling exhausted and anxious during the day. She also wrestled with feelings of guilt, constantly questioning if she could've prevented the accident. Psychologically, Jane began to exhibit symptoms of PTSD, such as flashbacks of the event and avoidance of anything that reminded her of the trauma, including the route she used to drive daily.

Case Study 2: Ahmed
Ahmed, a 45-year-old man, experienced chronic trauma in his childhood. Growing up in an abusive household, Ahmed was exposed to physical and emotional violence from a young age. This prolonged trauma impacted Ahmed's physical health, leading to stress-related conditions such as migraines and high blood pressure in his adult life. Emotionally, Ahmed struggled with forming intimate relationships, fearing the vulnerability they required. He had a pervasive feeling of worthlessness, often feeling undeserving of love or happiness. These feelings stemmed from the constant belittlement he faced as a child. Psychologically, Ahmed grappled with depression and complex PTSD, a condition often seen in individuals who've experienced chronic trauma. He had difficulty trusting people and experienced a sense of detachment from his own emotions, a coping mechanism developed during his traumatic childhood.

These two case studies illustrate how trauma can manifest differently depending on its nature (acute or chronic) and the individual's personal circumstances. Jane and Ahmed's stories also demonstrate how the effects of trauma can permeate various aspects of life, including physical health, emotional wellbeing, and psychological functioning. However, these stories should also serve as a reminder that while trauma can be devastating, it's possible to seek help, heal, and lead a fulfilling life.

Summary:
Trauma, an emotional response to distressing events, can result from a single incident like a car accident or prolonged situations like abuse or neglect. It can leave emotional scars and lead to feelings of fear, numbness, or reliving the traumatic event. However, it's important to remember trauma doesn't define you and healing is possible. Trauma can be classified as acute (resulting from a single event), chronic (multiple traumatic events over time), complex (multiple traumatic events, often during childhood), secondary or vicarious (experienced by those close to trauma survivors), historical or

collective (affecting entire communities), and developmental (early childhood trauma disrupting development). Trauma can impact physical health, emotional well-being, and psychological functioning. It can cause chronic health conditions, disrupt sleep patterns, lead to feelings of fear, sadness, guilt, anger, and shame, and result in psychological issues such as PTSD, anxiety disorders, and depression. Real-life cases, like Jane, who experienced acute trauma following a car accident, and Ahmed, who endured chronic trauma from childhood abuse, highlight the varied and profound impact of trauma. But they also underscore the possibility of recovery and resilience.

Key takeaways:
1. Understanding Trauma: Trauma can be described as an emotional response to distressing events that overwhelm a person's ability to cope. It can be a one-time event, a prolonged series of events, or chronic, repetitive experiences. Importantly, trauma is not about what's wrong with you, but what happened to you. It doesn't define you, but is part of your life's journey.
2. Types of Trauma: Trauma comes in various forms, including acute, chronic, complex, secondary or vicarious, historical or collective, and developmental trauma. Each type has unique characteristics, and a person can experience more than one type.
3. Effects of Trauma: Trauma leaves impacts on multiple levels: physical, emotional, and psychological. Physically, it can lead to health problems and disruptions in sleep or appetite. Emotionally, it might cause feelings like fear, sadness, guilt, anger, or shame, and lead to difficulties in relationships. Psychologically, it can lead to conditions such as PTSD, anxiety disorders, depression, and cognitive changes, disrupting a person's sense of safety and self-identity.
4. Personal Stories of Trauma: Through the case studies of Jane and Ahmed, we saw how trauma manifests differently in people's lives, highlighting the individual nature of trauma experiences and impacts.

It's crucial to remember that while trauma can have profound effects, it also opens avenues for growth, resilience, and transformation. The first step to healing is understanding, and by gaining knowledge about trauma, you're paving the way towards recovery. The subsequent chapters will provide more insights into the process of healing, offering tools and strategies to foster resilience and regain a sense of control over your life.

Chapter 2

Step 1 - Acceptance: Acknowledging Your Trauma

At its most basic, trauma is a deep emotional wound. It's a response to an intensely distressing event or series of events that shakes you to your core, making you feel threatened, helpless, or even fearing for your life. It's like a mental earthquake that disrupts the very ground you're standing on, leaving you feeling shaky, scared, and disoriented. Now, trauma isn't about everyday troubles. It's not about the fight you had with your spouse, or the stress of meeting work deadlines. Trauma is beyond the normal stressors we all face. It's about those events that are out of the ordinary, unexpected, and overwhelming. Think about the shock and disbelief you'd feel if you were in a serious car crash, or if you witnessed a horrific event. Imagine the deep pain and loss of losing someone you love in a sudden, tragic way. Or picture the fear and helplessness a child might feel while living in an abusive home. These are the kind of experiences we're talking about when we say trauma.

Trauma can also come from long-lasting, repeated events. For example, ongoing physical or emotional abuse, living in a war zone, or being subjected to bullying over a long period can all be traumatic. In these situations, it's not just one event but a series of distressing experiences that harm your emotional wellbeing. When you experience trauma, it can feel like your whole world has been turned upside down. You might find yourself having nightmares, or reliving the event in your mind. You could feel a constant sense of dread, or find it hard to trust others. It can disrupt your life, making you feel lost, confused, and alone. But remember, experiencing trauma isn't a sign of weakness. It means you've gone through something extraordinary and painful. Accepting and acknowledging your trauma is the first step towards healing. It's about saying, Yes, this happened to me. It was terrible, it hurt me, and it still affects me. This doesn't mean you're surrendering to it, but rather, you're starting to confront it. You're beginning to take control.

2.1: The Importance of Acceptance in Healing
Imagine trying to mend a broken bone without first acknowledging that it's broken. It would be not only painful but also detrimental to your overall healing. It's the same with emotional wounds. The first step to healing from trauma is acceptance - acknowledging the reality of the trauma you've experienced and recognizing its impact on your life. Trauma, in its essence, is a deep emotional wound that results from experiencing extremely distressing or disturbing events. Such events shatter your sense of security, leaving feelings of vulnerability, helplessness, and fear. This isn't about everyday stresses or problems; trauma stems from extraordinarily distressing situations that throw life off its normal rhythm.

Imagine surviving a natural disaster, or being in a severe car accident. Think of the profound loss felt when someone you love is abruptly taken from you. Consider the relentless distress experienced by a child living in a household filled with abuse. These experiences, whether a single event or repeated over time, encapsulate the essence of trauma. Experiencing trauma can make you feel as if your world has tilted on its axis. Your sleep might be disturbed by nightmares, or your days disrupted by flashbacks of the event. It's as if a shadow of dread constantly looms over you, coloring your worldview, and making trust a challenge. Understandably, this upheaval can lead to feelings of confusion, isolation, and despair. However, experiencing trauma doesn't mean you're weak. On the contrary, it means you've survived something incredibly challenging. You've been through an ordeal that has tested you, and here you are, standing, ready to start the process of healing.

Acceptance is a significant part of this healing process. It involves facing the reality of what happened, acknowledging that it was indeed traumatic, and allowing yourself to feel the pain that comes with it. Acceptance doesn't mean resignation; it's not about being okay with what happened or letting it define you. It's about giving yourself permission to recognize your suffering and validating your experience. This acknowledgment has a twofold purpose: First, it gives a name to your pain, which in itself can be empowering. It provides a context to your feelings, making them seem less overwhelming. Second, acceptance allows you to take ownership of your healing journey. By acknowledging your trauma, you're saying, Yes, this happened, and it hurt me, but I won't let it control me forever. Though trauma is painfully common, affecting people from all walks of life, the good news is that we, as humans, are inherently resilient. We have an innate capacity to heal, to bounce back from adversity, and to grow from our experiences. It's a testament to human strength that we can endure such hardships and not only survive but also pave the way for a future filled with hope and healing. Acceptance, as the first step in your journey towards healing, is not a sign of defeat but a mark of courage. It signifies your willingness to confront your pain, your readiness to seek help, and your resolve to move forward. Remember, acknowledging your trauma doesn't make you weak; it makes you a warrior. And as a warrior, you're taking the first stride on the path towards healing, strength, and resilience.

2.2: The Role of Denial in Trauma

Let's take a moment to talk about the elephant in the room, the shadowy presence that often accompanies trauma - Denial. It's a normal human reaction to pain and shock, a protective mechanism that shields us from the full impact of distressing events. When a traumatic experience strikes, denial is often our first line of defense. It's as if our minds, unable to fully grasp the enormity of what's happened, reject the reality of the situation to protect us from the onslaught of pain. Imagine you've stubbed your toe. Your initial response might be to dismiss the pain, maybe curse a bit, and then carry on. But as the pain persists, you're forced to acknowledge it and take action. In the case of trauma, this initial dismissal, this denial, can last much longer and can be much more profound.

But why do we fall into denial? Well, denial serves as a psychological band-aid, numbing us to the overwhelming pain that accompanies trauma. It's our psyche's attempt to maintain a semblance of normalcy, to keep the chaos at bay. It's as if our minds say, ""If I don't acknowledge the trauma, then it didn't really happen."" This form of self-protection can offer temporary relief, a sort of emotional buffer that buys us time to gradually process our experiences. However, when denial persists, it can become a stumbling block on the road to healing. Continuing to ignore or downplay your trauma can lead to emotional distress and potential mental health issues like anxiety, depression, or post-traumatic stress disorder (PTSD). Remaining in denial means you're still carrying that trauma around with you, its weight becoming an unseen burden that impacts your life and relationships.

Understandably, acknowledging your trauma can be an incredibly challenging and painful process. It involves pulling down the wall of denial and allowing the tide of emotions to wash over you. It means accepting that you've been hurt, that your experience was indeed traumatic, and that you are, rightfully so, affected by it. This is not an easy step, but it's a crucial one. Recognizing the role denial plays in your response to trauma is an integral part of the acceptance process. It's like turning on a light in a dark room; it helps you to see what's been hidden in the shadows. By bringing denial into the light, you can begin to understand its purpose and slowly start to peel away its layers. The denial you may be experiencing is not a sign of weakness or failure. It's a common reaction to trauma, an initial form of self-protection. But as you embark on your healing journey, it's important to gently challenge this denial, to bravely confront your pain and affirm your experience. This process of acknowledgment doesn't diminish your strength; instead, it showcases your courage. You're not alone in this journey, and through the path of acceptance, you're taking the first significant step towards healing, growth, and resilience.

2.3: Strategies for Coming to Terms with Your Trauma

At this point, you might be asking, "Okay, I recognize that I've experienced trauma and I understand the role of denial, but how do I actually come to terms with it? Let's dive into that.

When we talk about 'coming to terms' with trauma, we're really talking about integrating the reality of your experience into your life narrative. It's about moving from a place of denial and avoidance to acceptance and understanding, about shifting from feeling overwhelmed by your trauma to acknowledging it as part of your life's journey. But how do you make this transition? Here are some strategies:

a) **Identify your trauma:** This is about naming the traumatic event or experience and acknowledging its impact on you. It may be helpful to write down what happened, how it made you feel then, and how it's affecting you now. This can be a powerful exercise in validation and acknowledgement.

b) **Allow yourself to feel:** This can be the toughest part, but it's also essential. Denial often goes hand in hand with emotional numbness. As you let go of denial, you might start feeling a rush of emotions - and that's okay. It's important to allow these feelings to surface and to experience them without judgement.

c) **Practice self-compassion:** Remember, you didn't choose your trauma, and it's not a reflection of your worth or character. Be kind to yourself as you navigate this journey. Self-compassion might mean different things to different people - for you, it might involve self-care activities, positive self-talk, or simply giving yourself permission to take this process at your own pace.

d) **Seek support:** You don't have to do this alone. Reach out to trusted friends or family, join a support group, or consider seeking professional help. Connecting with others who understand what you're going through can be incredibly healing. It's also a reminder that you're not alone, and that it's okay to ask for help.

e) **Foster resilience:** Resilience is the capacity to bounce back from adversity, to adapt and grow in the face of challenges. Cultivating resilience might involve activities like meditation, exercise, creative pursuits, or engaging with nature. It's about finding healthy ways to cope and building a toolkit of strategies that you can draw on when times get tough.

There's no right or wrong way to go about this, and what works for one person might not work for another. That's okay. This is your journey, and it's about finding the path that feels right for you. Coming to terms with trauma is not a quick or easy process. It's a journey that takes time, patience, and courage. But as you take these steps, remember this: acknowledging your trauma doesn't make you weak, it makes you human. And it's the first step towards healing, growth, and a life that's defined not by your trauma, but by your resilience, strength, and capacity to bounce back better.

2.4: Activity: Self-Acceptance Journaling:
In understanding trauma, we must recognize that it's a deeply personal experience. It's not just an event that happens; it's a process that leaves an imprint on the mind and body. These imprints can linger, shaping how we view ourselves, others, and the world around us. So, it's crucial to acknowledge and understand our own personal trauma. One effective way to do this is through self-acceptance journaling. The concept of self-acceptance journaling stems from the recognition that healing from trauma is not just about moving past it, but also about fully accepting and integrating that part of your story. It's about acknowledging your experiences, your feelings, and the impact of the trauma on your life, but also recognizing your resilience and strength. Imagine your trauma as a book. Right now, it might feel like a book with chapters missing or pages torn out. It's a story that doesn't quite make sense, or a story that's too painful to read. Self-acceptance journaling is about gently filling in those pages, bringing clarity to your story, and, ultimately, helping you to accept it - not as a defining factor of who you are, but as a part of your life experience. To start, all you need is a notebook and pen. Find a quiet, comfortable place where you won't be disturbed. Write about the trauma you experienced. You don't have to dive into the most painful parts right away. Start wherever feels comfortable. As you write, try to describe not just what happened, but how it made you feel. This can help validate your experiences and emotions.

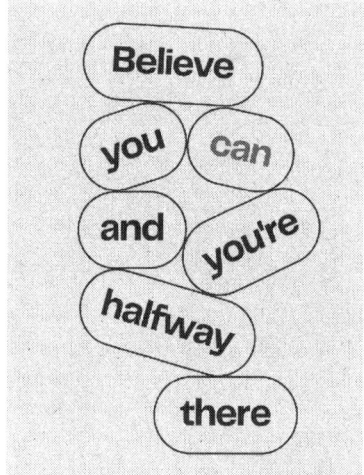

From there, consider writing about the impact the trauma has had on your life. This might include changes in your behavior, relationships, or self-perception. Again, this is not about blaming yourself or dwelling on the negative, but about understanding the role the trauma has played in your life. Next, write about your strengths and the ways you've shown resilience. Reflect on moments where you've managed to push through difficult times, or instances where you've shown courage, compassion, or strength. This part of journaling can help build your self-esteem and remind you of your capacity to cope. Over time, self-acceptance journaling can help you make sense of your experiences, affirm your feelings, and highlight your resilience. It's a way of saying, This is what happened to me, this is how it made me feel, and this is how I've grown from it. Your trauma is part of your story, but it doesn't define you. Through self-acceptance journaling, you can begin to understand and accept your trauma, while also recognizing your strength and resilience. And this is a crucial step on your path towards bouncing back better.

Summary:
Acceptance plays a pivotal role in the healing process as it allows for the acknowledgment of this pain and its impact on one's life. Denial is introduced as a natural reaction to trauma, acting as a psychological band-aid to temporarily shield us from pain. However, prolonged denial can hinder the healing process. Strategies such as

identifying trauma, allowing oneself to feel, practicing self-compassion, seeking support, and fostering resilience are shared to help readers come to terms with their trauma. An activity, Self-Acceptance Journaling, is provided as a therapeutic tool to explore and process trauma in a controlled, compassionate manner.

Key Takeaways:
1. Acceptance is the first step in healing trauma: Recognizing the reality of the trauma and its impact on your life is the first step towards healing.
2. Denial often accompanies trauma: Denial acts as an initial form of self-protection and can provide temporary relief, but long-term denial can hinder healing.
3. There are various strategies for coming to terms with trauma: These include identifying trauma, allowing oneself to feel, practicing self-compassion, seeking support, and fostering resilience.
4. Self-Acceptance Journaling can be a beneficial activity: It allows you to express your feelings, validate your experiences, and realize your resilience.
5. Trauma does not define you: While trauma is part of your life's journey, it doesn't define you. Recognizing your strength and resilience in the face of adversity is a crucial part of the healing process.

Chapter 3

Step 2 - Seek Support: Building Your Healing Network

When we find ourselves lost in the wilderness of our emotions after a traumatic event, it's easy to feel isolated and alone. However, it's crucial to understand that healing from trauma doesn't have to be a lonely journey. That's where Step 2 comes into play - seeking support and building your healing network. Think about it this way: if you had a deep cut on your hand, would you take care of it alone? Probably not. You'd likely seek help, perhaps from a doctor or a loved one. The same applies to emotional wounds. They may not be visible like a cut, but they are just as real and need care. Your healing network is your emotional 'first aid kit'. It can be made up of various individuals, groups, or resources. Maybe it's a close friend who's always there to listen, or a therapist who provides professional guidance. It could even be an online community of people who have experienced similar trauma.

Building your healing network is about reaching out, connecting with others, and letting them know that you could use a bit of help. It's about opening up to the love, kindness, and wisdom that's available around you, even if it doesn't seem like it sometimes. Seeking support is not a sign of weakness but a powerful step towards healing. It shows that you're committed to your journey of bouncing back better, ready to heal, and capable of embracing your inner strength.

3.1: The Role of Social Support in Trauma Recovery
When we go through traumatic experiences, we're like a boat tossed about in a stormy sea. The waves are huge, the wind is powerful, and it seems like we're all alone, trying to navigate through it all. But imagine if you had a crew on this boat, helping you handle the sails, anchor, and rudder. Wouldn't it be easier to navigate? That's what social support during trauma recovery is like—it's your crew, helping you navigate through the storm. One of the most vital roles of social support in trauma recovery is providing emotional comfort. When you share your pain, fears, and struggles with others who care about you, it lightens the emotional burden. They may not fully understand what you're going through, but their empathy, validation, and compassion can help soothe your emotional wounds.

Additionally, social support provides perspective. When we're in the middle of a traumatic experience, our thoughts can become clouded by negative emotions. Friends, family, or a therapist can help us see things from a different angle, reminding us that it's okay to grieve, it's okay to take time, and most importantly, it's okay to ask for help. In some cases, people who have experienced similar trauma can provide guidance and practical tips for coping. They've walked a similar path and can show you the way forward. This sense of shared experience can also foster a deeper connection and understanding, making you feel less alone in your journey. The role of social support isn't just about emotional comfort, perspective, or practical advice, though. It's also about reminding you of your strength and resilience. When we're in pain, we often forget how strong we actually are. The people in your healing network can help remind you of your inner strength, your courage, your progress, and your potential to heal and grow from this experience.

But remember, seeking and accepting social support is a two-way street. It requires courage and vulnerability to open up and share your experiences. It's okay if it feels scary or difficult at first; that's natural. Take it slow, start with someone you trust, and remember that it's okay to set boundaries. Finally, it's essential to keep in mind that everyone's healing journey is unique. What works for one person might not work for another. That's why it's crucial to build a diverse healing network that can provide different kinds of support. It can include close friends, family members, mental health professionals, support groups, online communities, or even self-help resources like this book. Social support plays a pivotal role in trauma recovery. It's your crew, helping you navigate through the storm. And with the right support, you can not only survive the storm but also learn how to sail your boat better for future voyages. It's a powerful testament to the human capacity for resilience, showing how we can bounce back better from even the most challenging experiences.

3.2: Identifying Your Support Network

Just as a garden grows best when it's nurtured by a diverse ecosystem, your healing journey thrives best when surrounded by a diverse support network. It's the different types of support from various sources that help you bounce back better. So how do you identify your support network? Let's explore that together:

Firstly, consider the people who make you feel safe, listened to, and valued. These are the people you trust, the ones you can confide in without fear of judgment or rejection. They could be close friends, family members, or even a trusted co-worker. It's not about the quantity of people but the quality of the relationship.

However, remember that not everyone in your close circle will be equipped to support you in the way you need. That's not a reflection on their love or care for you, but rather a recognition that everyone has their strengths and weaknesses. This is where professional support comes into the picture. Therapists, counselors, or psychiatrists have the training and experience to guide you through the healing process, offering strategies and tools that are based on scientific research. Apart from professional help, consider peer support groups. These groups consist of individuals who have experienced similar types of trauma. Being in such a group can offer a sense of belonging and understanding that's hard to find elsewhere. They can share their own experiences, coping strategies, and insights, helping you feel less alone and more hopeful about your journey. You can find these groups in your local community or online.

Your support network isn't only about people, though. Self-help books, online resources, podcasts, and workshops can provide invaluable insights and tools for healing.

They can help you understand your experiences better, offer coping strategies, and motivate you towards healing. Finally, don't forget to include yourself in your support network. Self-care and self-compassion are critical in healing from trauma. Learn to listen to your needs, be patient with your progress, and celebrate small victories. Remember, you are your own best friend and advocate in this journey. Identifying your support network might take some time, and it might require you to step out of your comfort zone, especially when it comes to seeking professional help or joining a support group. But remember, it's a step worth taking. Just like a boat needs a diverse crew to navigate the stormy sea effectively, you need a diverse support network to navigate your healing journey. To sum up, your support network is your healing ecosystem, made up of different types of support from various sources. It includes close relationships, professional help, peer support groups, self-help resources, and most importantly, self-care. Together, they create a nurturing environment that promotes growth, resilience, and healing. So take some time to identify your support network and don't be afraid to reach out for support. Remember, every step you take towards building your support network is a step towards bouncing back better.

3.3: How to Reach Out for Help

Asking for help can feel daunting, even scary, especially when you're dealing with trauma. It may feel like you're burdening others or exposing your vulnerability. However, reaching out for help is not a sign of weakness; it's a sign of strength and courage. It's an acknowledgment that you're ready to heal and grow, and that's incredibly powerful. So, how do you take this brave step? Let's walk through it together. The first step in reaching out for help is acknowledging your need for it. It might sound simple, but it's not always easy. Society often teaches us to be independent and self-reliant, but in this case, it's essential to remember that everyone needs help sometimes. There's no shame in that. Recognize your feelings and understand that it's perfectly okay to need support.

Next, identify who you want to reach out to. Maybe it's a trusted friend or family member. Perhaps it's a professional counselor or a support group. It's important to choose someone who you believe will be understanding and supportive. Keep in mind that different people can offer different types of support. It's okay to reach out to more than one person or group to ensure your needs are fully met. Once you've identified who to reach out to, plan what you want to say. It might be helpful to write down what you're feeling, what you're struggling with, and what kind of help you need. This step can help you articulate your thoughts and needs more clearly when you're ready to communicate them. When you're ready to reach out, choose a comfortable setting and approach the person respectfully and honestly. You might start by expressing your trust in them and then gradually share your feelings and struggles. Be specific about how they can help you, whether it's just listening, providing advice, or helping you find professional help. Remember, it's okay to express your needs clearly.

Reaching out for help also means being open to receiving it. It might not always come in the form you expect or from the person you expect. Be receptive to the support offered to you and remember that it's okay to decline help if it doesn't feel right for you. Finally, be patient with yourself and others. Remember, people might not always react as you expect them to, and that's more about them than you. Don't let any negative experiences discourage you from seeking the help you need. Reaching out for help is a critical step in your healing journey. It's an act of self-love and a testament to your resilience.

3.4: Case Study: Building a Support Network From Scratch

Meet Anna, a young woman who had to face severe trauma early in her life due to an accident that changed her world overnight. Anna's journey can offer us deep insights into the process of building a support network from scratch. When Anna first faced her trauma, she felt lost, scared, and alone. She was in a new city, far from her family, and felt disconnected from the world around her. She realized that to bounce back and start healing, she needed to reach out and build a support network. It was challenging, but Anna was determined. Anna's first step was to acknowledge her need for help. She came to terms with her trauma and allowed herself to feel the pain and the fear. She understood that healing was a journey she didn't have to embark on alone, and asking for help was not a sign of weakness but rather an act of courage and resilience. Next, she started identifying potential sources of support. Anna began by seeking professional help. She reached out to a local counselor who specialized in trauma healing. This professional guidance became an essential part of her support network, offering her tools and strategies to manage her emotional wounds. Alongside professional help, Anna sought emotional support. She joined a local support group for trauma survivors. Here, she met people who were experiencing similar struggles. They could understand what she was going through, and they shared their coping strategies, offering empathy, advice, and mutual support.

Anna also started reaching out to her friends. Initially, she feared judgment or pity, but she found that her fears were mostly unfounded. When she reached out, expressing her trust in them, and shared her struggles honestly, her friends were understanding and supportive. Additionally, Anna reconnected with her family, maintaining regular phone calls and visits when possible. Their emotional and practical support played a significant role in her recovery. She also used online resources and social media to connect with people worldwide who were going through similar experiences. She found virtual support groups, forums, and social media platforms that centered around trauma healing. These online connections provided additional layers of understanding and empathy. Throughout this journey, Anna experienced setbacks and challenges. Not everyone she reached out to was supportive or understanding. But she learned to focus on the positive responses and not to internalize any negative ones. She realized that her healing journey was her own, and she had the right to define who could be part of her support network. Building a support network from scratch wasn't easy for Anna, but it was instrumental in her healing journey. With time, patience, and persistence, she managed to create a circle of support that helped her navigate through her trauma and foster her inner strength. Anna's story reminds us that building a support network is possible, even from scratch, and it plays a vital role in bouncing back better from trauma.

Summary:

We explore the role of social support in trauma recovery, how to identify and reach out to your support network, and a practical case study of Anna, who built her support network from scratch. Healing from trauma is a challenging journey, but you don't have to go through it alone. Building a support network can provide emotional comfort, practical advice, and a sense of shared experience, helping you bounce back better.

Key Takeaways:
1. Building a diverse healing network plays a pivotal role in trauma recovery. It can provide emotional comfort, perspective, practical advice, and remind you of your strength and resilience.
2. Your support network can include close friends, family members, mental health professionals, support groups, online communities, and self-help resources. Don't forget to include yourself in this network.
3. Identifying your support network involves recognizing people who make you feel safe, listened to, and valued. Not everyone will be able to support you in the way you need, and that's okay.
4. Reaching out for help is an act of courage. It involves acknowledging your need for help, deciding who to reach out to, planning what you want to say, and being open to receiving help.
5. Building a support network from scratch may seem daunting, but it's possible. Like Anna's story, with time, patience, and persistence, you can create a network that supports your healing journey and fosters your inner strength.

Chapter 4

Step 3 - Self-Care: Prioritizing Your Well-being

Embracing self-care is a vital part of your journey towards healing from trauma. This means placing your well-being at the center and consciously dedicating time and effort to nurturing your mental, emotional, and physical health. Think of self-care as fuel for your recovery engine. When your tank is empty, the journey forward seems daunting and almost impossible. But when it's full, you have the energy and the resilience to navigate even the roughest terrains. Imagine self-care as a bubble bath, warm and inviting, filled with the things that replenish and renew you. It could be a leisurely walk in the park, immersing yourself in a good book, meditating, or simply enjoying a cup of tea. These activities may seem small, but their impact is significant. They create a refuge, a safe space where you can pause, breathe, and refuel.

Now, self-care isn't always easy or enjoyable. It also includes making tough choices, like setting boundaries, saying 'no' when needed, and seeking help when things get overwhelming. Remember, it's not about being selfish; it's about preserving your energy to better navigate your healing journey. And finally, be gentle with yourself in this process. You don't have to master self-care overnight. It's a practice, something you'll get better at over time. Start small, listen to your needs, and slowly build your unique self-care routine. Healing is a journey, and self-care is your loyal companion on this journey. Prioritizing your well-being isn't an indulgence, it's a necessity. So go ahead, fill your self-care tank, and take that next step forward in your journey!

4.1: Understanding Self-Care
When you're wounded emotionally, the aftermath is often marked by feelings of despair, fear, and a sense of being out of control. This is where self-care steps in as a beacon of hope and healing. Self-care for trauma involves recognizing that trauma disrupts your sense of self and well-being. You may feel disconnected from your body and emotions, and everything around you may seem overwhelming. This is normal. It's a protective response by your body. But it's also a sign that you need to gently shift your focus back to yourself. Trauma self-care starts with creating safety in your environment and within yourself. This could be through calming routines, quiet spaces, or safe relationships. A predictable routine, for instance, can help rebuild a sense of control and safety. From having regular meals to maintaining a consistent sleep schedule, these routines anchor you, providing comfort and structure in the chaos that trauma often brings. Next, self-care includes tuning into your body. Trauma can cause a disconnection from your physical self. Reconnecting can be as simple as breathing exercises, yoga, or mindful walking. These practices anchor you in the present moment, reminding you that you are here and you are safe. They also help in releasing trauma held in your body in a gentle, controlled manner.

Another significant aspect of self-care is managing triggers. These are stimuli that remind you of the traumatic event and can cause distress. Identifying these triggers and developing coping strategies is a vital self-care practice. For example, if crowded places make you anxious, a coping strategy could be to shop at off-peak hours or do online shopping. Emotional self-care is equally important. This involves expressing and validating your feelings without judgment. It could be through therapy, journaling, or art. Remember, it's okay to feel sad, angry, or scared. These emotions are part of the healing process. Finally, self-care involves reaching out for help when needed. You don't have to navigate your healing journey alone. Whether it's leaning on a trusted friend, joining a support group, or seeking professional help, reaching out is a testament to your strength. In essence, self-care in trauma is about recognizing and honoring your needs, setting boundaries, and taking steps towards nurturing your overall well-being. It's a journey of self-compassion, patience, and resilience. Remember, self-care isn't a luxury, it's a necessity on your path to heal from trauma and embrace your inner strength.

4.2: Physical Self-Care: Exercise, Sleep, and Nutrition
As we progress on the path of trauma healing, it's essential to understand the role of physical self-care. This encompasses three main pillars - exercise, sleep, and nutrition, all vital components of your overall health and well-being. Firstly, let's discuss exercise. In the face of trauma, it might feel challenging to engage in physical activity. However, even light exercise can make a significant difference. It doesn't mean you have to run a marathon or hit the gym daily. Simple activities like walking in nature, practicing yoga, or even stretching at home can help. The focus should be on moving your body in a way that feels good to you. Exercise helps release endorphins, often referred to as 'feel-good hormones.' It also aids in reducing stress and anxiety while promoting better sleep. Next is sleep, an often overlooked but critical aspect of physical self-care. Trauma can disrupt your sleep patterns, leading to insomnia or frequent nightmares. Prioritizing quality sleep becomes paramount in this context.

Establishing a sleep routine can help tremendously. This might include winding down before bed with a book, keeping screens away, ensuring a dark, quiet, and comfortable sleep environment. If sleep difficulties persist, consider seeking professional help. Remember, good sleep equates to better physical health and emotional resilience.
Lastly, let's delve into nutrition. What you consume plays a vital role in how you feel physically and emotionally. When dealing with trauma, it might be tempting to reach for comfort food, which is okay occasionally. However, it's essential to nourish your body with balanced meals. Include a variety of fruits, vegetables, whole grains, lean proteins, and healthy fats in your diet. Staying hydrated is equally important. Good nutrition fuels your body, supports your mood, and fosters a sense of well-being.

One essential point to note while discussing physical self-care is the idea of moderation and self-compassion. Some days, you might not feel up to exercising, or you might have a night of poor sleep, or you might indulge in comfort food. That's okay. Healing from trauma is not a linear journey, and there will be ups and downs. Physical self-care isn't about perfection; it's about consistently making efforts that favor your well-being. The significance of physical self-care cannot be overstated. Exercise, sleep, and nutrition form a triad that underpins your capacity to heal and bounce back from trauma. These elements nourish not just your body but also your mind and spirit. In prioritizing physical self-care, you aren't just surviving; you are fostering resilience, strength, and a sense of control that propels you towards a healthier, happier self. In the end, it's crucial to remember this: You are worthy of this care. You are worthy of feeling healthy, rested, and nourished.

4.3: Emotional Self-Care: Mindfulness, Emotional Regulation, and Leisure

As we continue our exploration into self-care, we now turn to emotional self-care, a key aspect of trauma healing. This concept involves three central elements: mindfulness, emotional regulation, and leisure. Let's start with mindfulness. At its core, mindfulness is about being present, consciously aware of your thoughts, feelings, and sensations without judgment. Practicing mindfulness can help you acknowledge and accept your emotions as they come, rather than suppress or avoid them. It's like taking a step back and observing your emotions from a distance. You could cultivate mindfulness through activities like meditation, deep-breathing exercises, or even mindful eating and walking. The aim here is to ground yourself in the present, providing a safe space to experience your emotions and thoughts.

Next, we delve into emotional regulation, the process of managing and responding to intense emotions. Trauma can sometimes make our emotions feel overwhelming, as if we're on a roller coaster with no end in sight. But emotional regulation strategies can provide us with tools to navigate these ups and downs. This might involve identifying triggers, learning to pause before reacting, or using coping strategies like journaling, talking to a trusted friend, or professional therapy. The objective is not to eliminate negative emotions, but to manage them in a way that they don't control your life. Lastly, we discuss the role of leisure in emotional self-care. This encompasses activities that bring you joy, relaxation, and fulfillment. Whether it's reading a book, painting, gardening, watching your favorite show, or simply sitting quietly in nature, leisure activities can act as a balm for your emotional well-being. They provide a break from stress, boost your mood, and rekindle your inner spark. The key here is to intentionally make time for activities you enjoy and give you a sense of peace.

However, remember that emotional self-care isn't a one-size-fits-all approach. What works for someone else might not work for you, and that's okay. It's about discovering and incorporating practices that resonate with you, making you feel emotionally nourished and grounded. Navigating through the process of emotional self-care might be challenging, especially when dealing with trauma. You might experience setbacks, but it's essential to treat yourself with kindness and patience. Emotional self-care is not a linear path or a quick fix; it's a journey of self-discovery and self-compassion. Ultimately, emotional self-care is about honoring your feelings, respecting your boundaries, and investing in activities that uplift your spirit. It's about remembering that your emotions are valid and that you deserve moments of joy and peace amidst the healing process.

4.4: Activity: Creating Your Personalized Self-Care Plan

Now that we've explored the concepts of physical and emotional self-care, it's time to apply them by creating your personalized self-care plan. This plan will serve as a go-to guide, helping you integrate self-care practices into your daily life.

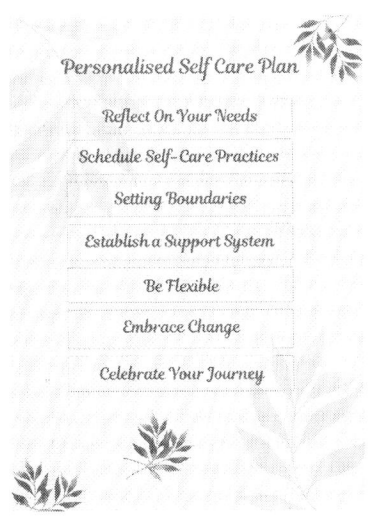

Personalised Self Care Plan
- Reflect On Your Needs
- Schedule Self-Care Practices
- Setting Boundaries
- Establish a Support System
- Be Flexible
- Embrace Change
- Celebrate Your Journey

1. **Reflect on Your Needs:**
Identify what rejuvenates you physically, emotionally, and mentally.
Understand that your self-care practices are unique and personal to you.

2. **Schedule Self-Care Practices:**
Incorporate small, manageable self-care habits into your daily routine.
Aim to make self-care a habitual practice, not an overwhelming task.

3. **Setting Boundaries:**
Learn to say 'no' to additional responsibilities when feeling overwhelmed.
Limit engagement with stress-inducing factors, like excessive social media usage.

4. **Establish a Support System:**
Include trusted friends, family members, or professionals like therapists or counselors in your journey.
Shared experiences can provide encouragement and empathy.

5. **Be Flexible:**
Understand that your self-care plan should serve you, not constrain you.
Be open to making necessary adjustments according to your current circumstances.

6. **Embrace Change:**
Be prepared to adapt your self-care plan as you evolve.
Don't hesitate to try new strategies and discard what isn't working.

7. **Celebrate Your Journey:**
Recognize each step towards self-care as a step towards healing.
Celebrate your progress and remind yourself of your resilience.

Crafting a personalized self-care plan is an ongoing process. It's about tuning into your needs, making conscious efforts to care for yourself, and navigating your journey with self-love and self-respect.

Summary:
Self-care involves both the mind and body, including aspects such as physical exercise,

sleep, nutrition, emotional mindfulness, emotional regulation, and leisure activities. It asserts that self-care is not a luxury but a necessity when recovering from trauma. The chapter also guides readers on creating a personalized self-care plan, highlighting the importance of setting boundaries, creating a support system, and being flexible to changing needs and circumstances.

Key Takeaways:
1. Self-care is an essential part of trauma recovery, focusing on nurturing mental, emotional, and physical health.
2. Physical self-care involves regular exercise, quality sleep, and balanced nutrition. It's about creating habits that promote physical well-being.
3. Emotional self-care includes mindfulness, emotional regulation, and engaging in leisure activities that bring joy and relaxation.
4. Trauma self-care begins with creating safety within oneself and in one's environment, managing triggers, expressing emotions without judgment, and reaching out for help when needed.
5. Creating a personalized self-care plan involves reflecting on individual needs, integrating self-care practices into daily routines, setting boundaries, and having a support system.
6. Flexibility is crucial in this plan as needs may change over time.
7. Healing from trauma is not a linear journey, and it's important to treat oneself with kindness and patience throughout the process.

Chapter 5

Step 4 - Therapy: Utilizing Professional Help

Seeking professional help in your journey of healing is not a sign of weakness. Rather, it signifies your strength and courage in facing your traumatic experiences. There are various kinds of therapists, such as psychologists, psychiatrists, or counselors, and each one of them is equipped with the tools and expertise to assist you in your healing journey. Therapy provides a safe space where you can openly express your thoughts, feelings, and fears without judgment. Therapists are trained to listen and offer guidance that's tailored to your unique situation. They employ different therapeutic techniques, such as cognitive-behavioral therapy (CBT), dialectical behavior therapy (DBT), or eye movement desensitization and reprocessing (EMDR) among others. These techniques are designed to help you understand and manage your emotions, change negative thinking patterns, and cope with trauma triggers.

Your therapist's office becomes a sanctuary where you can uncover layers of pain, giving voice to your silent screams. Within this sanctuary, you're guided gently towards insights and realizations, and you gain practical tools to cope with life's adversities. Over time, you'll learn to appreciate the beauty of vulnerability, as you find strength in your emotions and gradually rebuild your inner self. Remember, there's no 'one-size-fits-all' in therapy. What works for one might not work for another. The journey is personal and distinct. Patience is key. Healing takes time, but with each step, you move closer to a stronger, healthier you.

5.1: Why Therapy Matters
Sometimes life can throw a curveball that hits hard. These hits, in the form of traumatic events, can lead to emotional wounds that may fester and affect our daily functioning. This is where therapy becomes crucial, serving as a vital tool to help us understand, address, and heal from our traumatic experiences. One might wonder, why therapy? Can't we just talk to a friend or family member? While having a strong support system is undoubtedly important, there are aspects of professional therapy that set it apart. Therapists possess the necessary training to navigate our complex emotional landscapes. They can identify unhealthy patterns, behaviors, or beliefs that we might overlook, offering us guidance and strategies to overcome these obstacles.

In the aftermath of trauma, we might find ourselves stuck in patterns of avoidance, self-blame, or hyperarousal. Therapy provides a non-judgmental space to examine these responses and to explore healthier ways to cope. It equips us with tools to break free from these patterns, helping us regain control and ownership of our lives. Additionally, trauma can sometimes lead to feelings of isolation and disconnect. Therapy provides a space of connection and validation. When we share our stories, feelings, and fears in therapy, we're met with understanding and acceptance. This experience can be incredibly healing, reinforcing that we're not alone in our struggles. Therapy also aids in understanding the roots of our trauma. By shedding light on the underlying causes, we can develop a more compassionate view of ourselves. We learn that our reactions and feelings are natural responses to unnatural events. This understanding can help reduce self-blame and cultivate self-compassion, integral parts of healing.

The exploration in therapy doesn't stop at the past; it extends into our future as well. Therapy supports us in building resilience, teaching us ways to better respond to future stressors or adversities. We learn to manage our emotions, enhance our coping skills, and nurture our inner strength, all of which empower us to bounce back better from future challenges. Moreover, the benefits of therapy seep into various aspects of our lives. It can improve our relationships as we gain a better understanding of ourselves and how we interact with others. It can enhance our performance at work or school by improving our concentration, motivation, and overall mental well-being. Lastly, therapy provides a safe space for self-expression and emotional release. Expressing our emotions can be a cathartic experience, releasing pent-up feelings and promoting emotional balance. The act of sharing our stories can be empowering, giving voice to our experiences and reminding us of our strength and resilience.

As we navigate the path of healing from trauma, therapy can be our guiding light, illuminating our way forward. While the journey isn't always easy, the rewards are significant: a deeper understanding of ourselves, healthier coping mechanisms, stronger relationships, and a resilient spirit ready to face life's challenges. Remember, seeking help isn't a sign of weakness; it's a testament to our courage and resilience. In the following sections, we'll delve into how to choose a therapist and what to expect from therapy, to help you make the most of this crucial step in your healing journey.

5.2: Types of Therapeutic Approaches for Trauma
When it comes to healing from trauma, there are many different types of therapeutic approaches available, each with its unique strengths. While all therapies aim to help you heal, the right one for you depends on your specific needs, circumstances, and personal comfort. Let's explore some of the most common approaches used in trauma therapy. Cognitive Behavioral Therapy (CBT) is a widely-used method that helps you understand how your thoughts influence your feelings and behaviors. It helps you identify and challenge negative or unhelpful thought patterns that might have formed due to your trauma. You learn to replace these thoughts with healthier, more positive ones, enabling you to cope better with life's challenges. Eye Movement Desensitization and Reprocessing (EMDR) is another effective method for trauma. In EMDR, you're guided to recall traumatic events while generating side-to-side eye movements. This process helps reduce the intensity of your traumatic memories and changes how these memories affect you. It's like reprogramming your brain's response to trauma.

Dialectical Behavior Therapy (DBT) is a form of therapy that focuses on teaching you skills to manage your emotions, improve your relationships, and tolerate distress. This therapy can be particularly helpful if your trauma has led to intense emotional reactions or if you struggle with self-destructive behaviors. Exposure Therapy is a type of therapy where you're gradually and repeatedly exposed to thoughts, feelings, and situations that remind you of the trauma. This helps you reduce fear and anxiety and improve your coping abilities. The idea is that through repeated exposure, your trauma-related reactions lessen over time. Another popular therapeutic approach is Somatic Therapy. This therapy focuses on the connection between the body and the mind. It helps you release the physical tension or stress that's often stored in your body after a traumatic event. By focusing on bodily sensations, you learn to release this stored trauma and heal.

Narrative Therapy can also be beneficial. This approach helps you tell the story of your trauma and separate yourself from it, helping you understand that you are not defined by your traumatic experiences. It's about reclaiming your life's narrative and recognizing your resilience. Art Therapy uses creative activities like drawing, painting, or collage-making to express and process traumatic memories. It provides a non-verbal outlet for emotions and can help you gain a new perspective on your experiences. These are just a few of the many therapeutic approaches available for trauma. Each person is unique, and what works for one might not work for another. That's why it's important to find a therapist with whom you feel comfortable, and who is trained in the approach that best suits your needs. Healing from trauma is a journey. It takes time, patience, and a lot of self-compassion. But with the right support and therapeutic approach, you can overcome your trauma, bounce back stronger, and live a fulfilling life. The next sections will guide you on how to choose a therapist and make the most out of your therapy sessions.

5.3: How to Choose the Right Therapist for You
Choosing a therapist can feel like finding a needle in a haystack. There are so many names, specialties, and approaches to choose from. How do you know who's the right one for you? Here are some practical tips to help you find the therapist that fits your needs and will guide you in your healing journey. Think of your first consideration as a practical one. You need to find someone who fits your budget, schedule, and location. Some therapists may offer sliding-scale fees, which means they adjust their charges based on your income. Consider if you'd prefer online or face-to-face sessions. Does

the therapist's working hours align with your schedule? These are important questions to get out of the way initially.

Next, consider their qualifications and specialties. It's important to choose a therapist who has specific experience and training in trauma therapy. Check if they have certifications in the types of therapy that you're interested in, such as Cognitive Behavioral Therapy (CBT), Eye Movement Desensitization and Reprocessing (EMDR), or Somatic Therapy. Personal comfort is crucial. You need to feel comfortable with your therapist - you'll be sharing your deepest thoughts and experiences with them. Some people might prefer a therapist of a specific gender, age, or cultural background, and that's entirely okay. You could also consider their communication style. Do you want someone who's more talkative and directive or someone who listens more and guides subtly? Professional reputation can also guide your decision. Look for reviews or ask for recommendations from people you trust. It can be reassuring to know that others have had positive experiences with the therapist you're considering.

Then comes the most important part: the 'therapeutic relationship'. Research shows that a good relationship between you and your therapist is one of the most important factors in successful therapy. When you meet your potential therapist for the first time, pay attention to your gut feelings. Do you feel heard, respected, and understood? Do you feel safe and comfortable? These are signs that you could build a strong therapeutic relationship. Lastly, don't be afraid to shop around. It's okay to meet with a few therapists before deciding on the right one for you. Most therapists understand this and offer an initial consultation to discuss your needs and their approach. This gives you a chance to see if you 'click' with them. It's completely fine to change therapists if you don't feel the current one is working for you, even after a few sessions. It's essential that you find someone who's a good fit for you and your needs. The journey to heal from trauma can be challenging, but having the right therapist by your side can make a world of difference.

5.4: Making the Most Out of Therapy: Tips and Strategies
Once you've found the right therapist, the next step is to ensure you're making the most of your therapy sessions. Just like a journey, getting the most out of therapy involves

preparation, active participation, and reflection. Here are some tips and strategies to guide you:

Be Open and Honest: Share your deepest thoughts, feelings, and fears without judgment. The more honest you are, the better your therapist can understand you and guide you. There's no right or wrong thing to say in therapy.

Active Participation: Therapy requires your active involvement, which might include facing painful memories, trying new behaviors, or practicing skills learned in therapy in your daily life.

Ask Questions: If you don't understand something, ask your therapist to explain it. If you're curious about a specific therapeutic approach, inquire about it.

Set Goals: Set clear goals with your therapist to give your therapy direction and help measure your progress. Goals can be big or small, like learning a new coping skill, improving a relationship, or working through a traumatic memory.

Practice Self-Care: Therapy can bring up intense emotions, so it's essential to practice self-care between sessions. This could involve activities such as going for a walk, journaling, meditating, or spending time with loved ones.

Reflect on Your Sessions: After each session, take some time to think about what you discussed, how you felt, and what you learned. Reflection can help you process your therapy and see how far you've come.

Communicate with Your Therapist: If something isn't working in your therapy, discuss it with your therapist. They're there to help you, and your feedback can help them tailor the therapy to better suit your needs.

Be Patient: Healing from trauma doesn't happen overnight; it's a journey with potential bumps along the way. Healing isn't linear, and even small steps forward count.

Embrace the Process: Therapy can be a powerful tool in your trauma healing journey. With openness, active participation, and patience, it can lead to profound change.

Summary:

Choosing the right therapist is a crucial step in the healing journey. Factors to consider include practical aspects like fees and availability, the therapist's qualifications and specializations, personal comfort, professional reputation, and the potential for a strong therapeutic relationship. It's perfectly fine to meet with a few therapists before settling on the right one for you. Once you've found a therapist, maximizing the benefits of therapy involves being open and honest, actively participating, setting clear goals, practicing self-care, reflecting on your sessions, and maintaining communication with your therapist. Remember, healing takes time, and patience is key.

Key Takeaways:

1. Therapy is a vital tool in the healing journey from trauma.
2. Choosing the right therapist involves several considerations, including qualifications, comfort, and a good therapeutic relationship.
3. Maximizing therapy benefits involves active participation, clear goal setting, self-care, and continuous reflection.
4. Patience is essential in the healing process.

Chapter 6

Step 5 - Expression: Releasing Your Emotions

"Expression: Releasing Your Emotions." This step is all about letting out those intense emotions you've been holding in, which is a vital part of healing from trauma. Think of your emotions as a pressure cooker. When you keep the lid on, the pressure builds. If not released, it could lead to an explosion. Similarly, when you suppress your emotions, they can intensify, often leading to stress, anxiety, or even physical health issues. So, it's crucial to find healthy outlets for your emotions. Expressing your emotions doesn't mean you need to have a big, dramatic outburst. It can be as simple as talking to someone you trust about how you're feeling, writing in a journal, or even creating art. It's about acknowledging your feelings, letting them out, and saying, "I see you, I feel you, and it's okay."

It's important to remember that all emotions, whether they're happy, sad, or somewhere in between, are part of the human experience. There's no such thing as a 'bad' emotion. In this chapter, we'll explore various ways to express your emotions, why it's important, and how it can help you heal from trauma and bounce back stronger. You'll find that releasing your emotions can be liberating, making room for more positive feelings and peace of mind.

6.1: The Importance of Emotional Expression:

The emotional expression is not only beneficial, but it is necessary. It is as vital to our wellbeing as eating or sleeping. Often, when we experience trauma, our initial instinct may be to suppress or avoid the difficult feelings associated with it. You might even have been told at times that it's better to be strong and keep your emotions to yourself. But burying these emotions doesn't make them disappear. They are still there, lurking beneath the surface, possibly manifesting as physical symptoms or exacerbating stress and anxiety. By expressing our emotions, we acknowledge them, which is the first step towards healing. We validate our feelings, showing ourselves that it's okay to feel this way. This can be a tremendous relief, lifting the burden of carrying these unexpressed feelings inside us. It allows us to face our emotions rather than fear them.

Moreover, expressing our emotions can lead to improved relationships. When we let others know how we feel, we create opportunities for understanding, empathy, and deeper connections. It makes us human, authentic, and relatable. But emotional expression is not just about releasing negative emotions. It's also about expressing positive feelings such as happiness, joy, and gratitude. By actively recognizing and expressing these positive emotions, we can foster a sense of positivity and resilience that helps in our recovery. When we express our emotions, we also gain a better understanding of ourselves. We start to see patterns in our emotional responses and can work towards managing our emotions better. For instance, you might notice that certain situations trigger feelings of anger or sadness, and acknowledging this can help you develop strategies to cope.

Another important aspect of emotional expression is its potential to provide relief and decrease the intensity of our feelings. When emotions are expressed, they lose some of their power over us. This process can also help in diffusing stress, calming the mind, and promoting physical health. There are several ways to express emotions, and different methods work for different people. Some may find solace in talking to a friend or family member, while others may prefer writing in a journal, painting, or even dancing. There is no 'right' way to express your emotions. It's about finding what works for you, a method where you feel safe and comfortable.

6.2: Healthy Ways to Express Your Emotions:
Now that we've explored the significance of emotional expression in the healing process, let's look at some healthy ways to express your emotions. Remember, there's no 'right' or 'wrong' way to express emotions. What matters is that the method you choose is safe, comfortable, and beneficial to you.

a) Verbal Expression: Speaking with a trusted friend, family member, or therapist can be incredibly healing. Sometimes, just voicing your feelings can take a weight off your shoulders. By verbalizing your emotions, you validate them and make them tangible, which often makes them easier to deal with.

b) Journaling: Writing about your feelings can be as therapeutic as speaking about them. It's a private space where you can be entirely honest and not worry about judgment. Journaling helps you recognize patterns in your emotions, which can be very helpful in managing your emotional health.

c) Artistic Expression: Creativity can be a wonderful outlet for emotions. Painting, drawing, sculpting, dancing, or making music allows you to express your feelings in non-verbal, yet powerful ways. Artistic expression can give voice to emotions that might be too complex or overwhelming to articulate in words.

d) Physical Activity: Exercise can be an excellent outlet for emotions, particularly those that induce high energy like anger or frustration. Engaging in physical activities such as running, yoga, or even just taking a walk, can help you channel these emotions healthily and reduce their intensity.

e) Meditation and Mindfulness: These practices encourage you to sit with your emotions without judgment. They teach you to observe your feelings and thoughts as they are, fostering a better understanding of your inner emotional landscape. This acceptance and awareness can lead to a healthier relationship with your emotions.

f) Crying: Despite societal norms that often label crying as a sign of weakness, it's a natural and healthy way to express emotions. Crying can bring a sense of relief, reduce stress, and help you cope with pain.

g) Expressing Through Actions: This could involve small acts of kindness for others when you're feeling grateful or happy. Conversely, when feeling sad or overwhelmed, you might express this by taking time off for self-care.

h) Therapy: Therapists provide a safe, confidential, and non-judgmental space for you to explore and express your emotions. They can offer techniques and tools to help you navigate your feelings effectively.

Lastly, remember it's okay to ask for help. If expressing your emotions feels overwhelming, reach out to a professional who can guide you through this journey. Healthy emotional expression is a skill that can be learned and honed over time. By practicing, you'll not only help yourself heal from past traumas but also build a strong foundation for better emotional health in the future.

6.3: Activity: Art Therapy - Drawing Your Emotions:
Art, in its many forms, is a universal language that can express what words often can't. It enables us to communicate our feelings and experiences in a way that can be profoundly healing. For this activity, we're going to focus on drawing. You don't need to be an artist or have drawing skills for this. It's about the process, not the outcome. For this you need a piece of paper and a set of colored pencils, crayons, or markers.

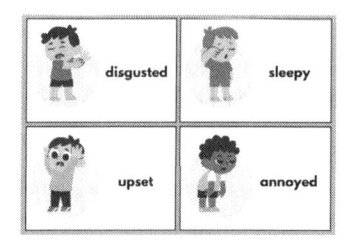

Step 1: **Choosing Your Emotion:** Think about a specific emotion that you've been feeling lately, one that's prominent in your mind. It could be sadness, anger, fear, joy, confusion, or anything else that's been lingering in your thoughts and feelings.

Step 2: **Visualization:** Close your eyes and give yourself a moment to feel this emotion deeply. What color does this emotion bring to mind? Does it have a shape? Is it heavy or light, sharp or soft? Visualize your emotion as completely as you can.

Step 3: **Putting it on Paper:** Open your eyes and begin to draw. Let your hand move freely. You might start with the color or shape that came to mind when you visualized your emotion. Don't worry about creating a masterpiece; just focus on representing your feelings on the paper in front of you.

Step 4: **Free Expression:** Allow yourself to be swept up in the act of drawing. If your emotion changes, change the colors or shapes you're using. If the emotion becomes intense, let your strokes become intense too. The paper is your safe space to express whatever you're feeling.

Step 5: **Reflection:** Once you feel that your drawing is complete, take a step back. Look at your work and reflect on the process. How did it feel to represent your emotion visually? Did anything surprise you? Did the process change how you felt about the emotion?

This activity isn't just about drawing; it's about giving your emotions a voice and an outlet. By doing this, you're acknowledging your feelings, making them tangible and, in a way, easier to understand. It's a process of validation and exploration, a journey of emotion and healing through creativity. Remember, the goal here is not to produce a beautiful piece of artwork but to give your emotions a physical form. Each color, each line, and each shape you create is a part of your emotional narrative, a step towards understanding yourself better. So keep drawing, keep expressing, and most importantly, keep healing.

6.4: Case Study: Healing Through Expressive Writing:

Anna, a 30-year-old graphic designer, experienced a traumatic event that left her emotionally scarred. She felt overwhelmed by feelings of sadness, anger, and confusion. She had trouble articulating her emotions verbally, and they seemed to be consuming her from the inside. In search of healing, Anna came across the concept of expressive writing. She had always enjoyed writing in her spare time, but she had never considered it as a potential pathway to emotional healing. She started with small steps, writing just a few lines every day. At first, the words on the page seemed disconnected, mirroring her state of mind. But as she persisted, she found her thoughts starting to untangle, becoming clearer as they took shape on paper. Anna's writing became a dialogue with herself. Some days, she wrote about her trauma, bringing forth the painful details that she had been unable to speak out loud. Other days, she wrote about her emotions, describing the heaviness of her sadness or the heat of her anger. She gave voice to her fears, hopes, and dreams. The pages of her notebook became a mirror of her inner world.

As Anna continued to express her feelings, she noted a shift within herself. The overwhelming emotions began to feel more manageable. The act of writing gave her a sense of control, an anchor in the storm of her emotions. She started understanding her feelings better, and this understanding paved the way for acceptance. Over time, she also began to notice patterns. She could identify triggers that intensified her emotional turmoil and patterns in her thought processes that were counterproductive. She was then able to work on changing these patterns, transforming her narrative gradually. Through expressive writing, Anna found a safe space for her emotions. It was a process that required her to be open, honest, and vulnerable with herself. It was challenging, but it was also liberating. She found herself able to let go of some of the pain that she had been holding on to. She found herself beginning to heal. This case study illustrates the therapeutic potential of expressive writing. Just like Anna, many individuals can benefit from such a practice. Expressing your emotions through writing can provide an outlet for your feelings, leading to a greater understanding and acceptance of your emotions. It allows you to confront your feelings in your own time, at your own pace, and in your own words.

Summary:
It highlights that emotional expression is not limited to negative emotions but also includes positive ones, leading to improved relationships, self-understanding, and relief from intense feelings. It includes an activity called "Art Therapy - Drawing Your Emotions," where individuals are encouraged to draw their emotions as a form of self-expression. It also presents a case study of Anna, who found healing through expressive writing. Anna discovered that writing allowed her to untangle her thoughts, understand her emotions better, and gain a sense of control over her emotional turmoil. Through the process, she experienced acceptance and gradual healing.

Key takeaways:
1. Emotional expression is essential for healing from trauma, as suppressed emotions can lead to negative consequences.
2. Expressing emotions, both positive and negative, fosters self-understanding, improved relationships, and relief from intense feelings.
3. Various healthy ways to express emotions include verbal expression, journaling,

artistic expression, physical activity, meditation, crying, expressing through actions, and seeking therapy.

4. Art therapy, such as drawing emotions, can be a powerful tool for self-expression and healing.

5. Expressive writing can provide an outlet for emotions, leading to greater understanding and acceptance of one's feelings.

6. Emotional expression is a skill that can be learned and developed over time, and seeking professional help is encouraged if the process feels overwhelming.

Chapter 7

Step 6 - Mindfulness: Cultivating Presence

Mindfulness is like an anchor, tethering you firmly to reality. It cultivates an inner peace that allows you to better process your experiences, especially when facing adversity or trauma. As you become more mindful, you become more aware of your emotions, thoughts, and actions without judging them, fostering a kinder relationship with yourself. Think of mindfulness as being a compassionate observer to your own life. By consciously paying attention to your thoughts and emotions, you gradually become less entangled in them. This can provide a healing balm to emotional wounds, as you're no longer endlessly replaying past hurts or fretting over future uncertainties.

This chapter will walk you through practical exercises and techniques to embed mindfulness into your daily life. We'll explore breathing exercises, mindfulness meditation, and mindful activities that can be seamlessly incorporated into your routines. Remember, mindfulness is not about achieving a state of perpetual happiness or tranquility, but about embracing life in all its complexities. It's about creating space for everything - joy, sadness, fear, and love - and acknowledging that these experiences, too, are part of the human condition. This understanding can fortify your inner strength, helping you bounce back better from life's challenges.

7.1: What is Mindfulness?

To understand the healing journey, one needs to appreciate the art of mindfulness. But, what exactly is mindfulness? The term might seem enigmatic, wrapped up in complex philosophies, but it's quite the opposite. It's a simple, yet profound concept: the practice of being present in the moment. Mindfulness, at its core, is about paying attention. It's about tuning into the symphony of life around you and within you, not getting lost in the whirl of thoughts, worries, and stresses that often dominate our minds. It's about experiencing life as it happens, rather than viewing it through the lens of our past or future.

Imagine you're walking in a park. The sun is warming your skin, the wind is rustling the leaves, and birds are singing their songs. But, your mind is elsewhere – you're worrying about a presentation you have to give tomorrow or ruminating over a conversation you had yesterday. You're physically in the park, but mentally, you're somewhere else entirely. This is where mindfulness comes in. Mindfulness would have you truly in the park. You would feel the sun on your skin, listen to the rustle of the leaves, hear the birds' songs, and notice the aroma of fresh earth. Your thoughts might still wander – that's just what minds do – but with mindfulness, you gently bring your attention back to the present moment.

But mindfulness isn't just about appreciating pleasant experiences. It's also about facing the uncomfortable ones. When feelings of sadness, anger, or fear arise, our instinct is often to push them away. Mindfulness, however, teaches us to hold space for these feelings. It encourages us to sit with the discomfort, to acknowledge it, but not to let it control us. This ability to sit with our emotions can be a powerful tool in trauma healing. We often store our traumatic experiences deep within, trying to forget them or minimize their impact. However, they have a way of surfacing, sometimes in disruptive and harmful ways. Mindfulness helps us process these experiences in a healthy, non-judgmental manner. By observing our emotions and thoughts without judgment, we can start to detach from them. This doesn't mean we ignore or negate them; instead, we observe them as temporary states, not defining truths. Anxious thoughts or feelings of sadness become just that—thoughts and feelings. They are not us, and they do not have to define our reality.

Mindfulness also promotes self-compassion. By becoming aware of our internal dialogue, we can start to challenge and change negative self-talk. We can learn to treat ourselves with the same kindness and understanding we would offer a good friend. This shift towards self-compassion can significantly aid the healing process, helping us to bounce back better from the challenges life throws at us. Mindfulness is a simple concept, but it's not always easy. It takes practice. Like strengthening a muscle, the more we use mindfulness, the stronger our ability to stay present becomes. But the rewards are plentiful—greater peace, understanding, and resilience, to name a few.

7.2: The Role of Mindfulness in Trauma Recovery:
So, how does mindfulness play a role in recovering from trauma? Traumatic experiences can leave deep emotional scars. Often, we might find ourselves trapped in the pain of the past or the fear of the future. This is where mindfulness offers a transformative tool for trauma recovery. Grounding in the Present: Trauma often makes us feel disconnected from the world around us. We may feel stuck in a moment of time, continually reliving painful experiences. Mindfulness helps ground us in the present moment, breaking the cycle of past and future ruminations. It doesn't erase the trauma, but it provides an anchor to the 'here and now.'
a) Observing without Judgment: With mindfulness, we learn to observe our thoughts and emotions without judgment. We start to see our feelings as they truly are - transient states that come and go. This detached observation can lessen the power trauma holds over us. We can acknowledge our pain without letting it define us.
b) Creating Space for Healing: Through mindfulness, we create a space for healing to occur. By acknowledging our pain, we make the first steps towards dealing with it. We bring our wounds out of the shadows and into the light. This can be uncomfortable at first, but it's a crucial step towards recovery.
c) Enhancing Self-Compassion: Mindfulness fosters self-compassion, encouraging us to treat ourselves with kindness and understanding. We begin to see that we're not at fault for our trauma, reducing feelings of guilt or self-blame. This shift can have a profound impact on our healing journey.
d) Building Resilience: Mindfulness not only helps us cope with our past traumas but also equips us with the tools to better handle future challenges. By cultivating

mindfulness, we build a resilience that helps us bounce back from life's difficulties more effectively.

e) Reducing Stress: Mindfulness has been shown to reduce stress, a common aftermath of trauma. It does this by promoting a relaxation response, a state of deep rest that changes our physical and emotional responses to stress. This can lead to improved mental well-being and an enhanced quality of life.

f) Improving Physical Health: Trauma can have physical implications as well, such as sleep disorders, chronic pain, and other stress-related ailments. Regular mindfulness practice can improve these conditions by fostering better sleep, reducing pain levels, and boosting overall health.

g) Promoting Connection: Lastly, mindfulness can help us reconnect with ourselves and others. Trauma can lead to feelings of isolation and detachment. Mindfulness helps us see that we are not alone in our experiences, promoting a sense of shared humanity. Mindfulness is not a magic bullet, but it is a powerful tool in your healing toolbox. As you learn to live more fully in the present, to observe without judgment, to hold space for your pain, and to cultivate self-compassion, you'll find yourself gaining strength and resilience. This strength will carry you forward, helping you not just to recover from your trauma, but to bounce back better!

7.3: Mindfulness Exercises for Healing Trauma:

Mindfulness might sound like a broad concept, but it's a skill that can be honed with practice. Here are some practical mindfulness exercises that can be powerful aids in your trauma healing journey:

1. Mindful Breathing: The simplest and most accessible tool for practicing mindfulness is your breath. When feeling overwhelmed, take a moment to focus solely on your breathing. Notice the sensation of the air entering and leaving your nostrils or the rise and fall of your chest. If your mind wanders, gently bring it back to the breath. Even just a few minutes of mindful breathing can create a calm oasis in the midst of chaos.

2. Body Scan: This exercise involves paying close attention to different parts of your body, from your toes to the top of your head. Lie down in a comfortable position and slowly bring your attention to each part of your body. Notice any sensations you feel, such as tension, warmth, or tingling, without trying to change anything. This can help

ground you in the present and foster a deeper connection with your body.

3. Mindful Walking: If you find sitting meditation challenging, try mindful walking. As you walk, focus on the sensation of your feet touching the ground, the rhythm of your steps, the movement of your arms. Take note of the sights, sounds, and smells around you. Mindful walking can be an excellent way to integrate mindfulness into your everyday life.

4. Loving-Kindness Meditation: This practice involves sending wishes of love, peace, and happiness to yourself and others. Start by sending these wishes to yourself, then to a loved one, then to someone neutral, then to someone you have difficulty with, and finally to all beings everywhere. This can enhance feelings of compassion and reduce feelings of isolation and anger.

5. Mindful Journaling: Writing can be a powerful outlet for processing emotions. Try to write about your experiences in a nonjudgmental way, focusing on your feelings in the present moment. Don't worry about grammar or punctuation - this is for you and you alone.

6. Mindful Eating: Eating is something we often do on autopilot. Try eating a meal mindfully, paying attention to the taste, texture, and smell of the food. Notice the sensation of the food in your mouth and the process of chewing and swallowing. This can be a powerful exercise in staying present.

7. Yoga and Mindful Movement: Yoga combines physical postures, breathing exercises, and meditation, making it a holistic practice for mindfulness. However, any form of mindful movement, even simple stretching, can help bring your attention back to the present.

Keep in mind that the goal of these exercises is not to erase or suppress your trauma. Instead, they're meant to help you create a safe space where you can observe your experiences without judgment. As you grow in your mindfulness practice, you may find it easier to navigate the healing journey, building resilience, and inner strength that will help you bounce back better.

7.4: Activity: Step by Step Guided Mindfulness Meditation:

Practicing mindfulness meditation can be a vital step in your trauma healing journey. Here's a simple, guided mindfulness meditation you can try at home. Remember, there's no right or wrong way to meditate. What matters most is your dedication to the practice and your compassion towards yourself during the process:

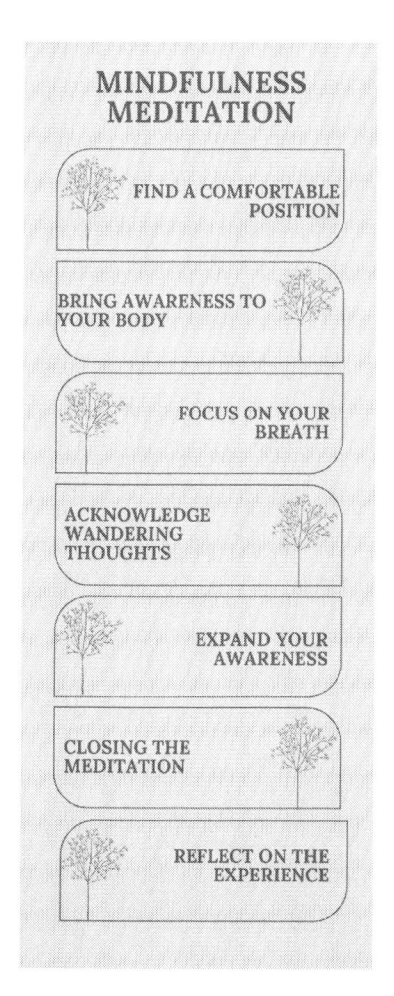

MINDFULNESS MEDITATION
- FIND A COMFORTABLE POSITION
- BRING AWARENESS TO YOUR BODY
- FOCUS ON YOUR BREATH
- ACKNOWLEDGE WANDERING THOUGHTS
- EXPAND YOUR AWARENESS
- CLOSING THE MEDITATION
- REFLECT ON THE EXPERIENCE

Step 1: Find a Comfortable Position

Find a quiet, comfortable place where you won't be disturbed for a few minutes. You can sit on a chair or cushion, with your feet flat on the floor and your spine upright but not stiff. You can also lie down if that's more comfortable. Close your eyes if you feel comfortable doing so, or keep them half-open, gazing softly downwards.

Step 2: Bring Awareness to Your Body

Bring your awareness to your physical body, noticing how it feels. Feel the weight of your body on the chair or floor. Notice the touch of your clothes against your skin, the temperature of the room. If there's tension in any part of your body, acknowledge it but don't try to change anything.

Step 3: Focus on Your Breath
Now, turn your attention to your breath. Notice the sensation of the breath as it enters and exits your nostrils or the rise and fall of your chest or abdomen as you breathe. You don't need to change your breathing in any way - just observe it.

Step 4: Acknowledge Wandering Thoughts
Your mind will likely wander—that's perfectly okay. When you notice it, gently acknowledge it and bring your attention back to your breath. This isn't a sign of failure, but a part of the process. It's the act of returning your focus that builds your mindfulness muscle.

Step 5: Expand Your Awareness
Once you're settled into the rhythm of your breath, expand your awareness to include your entire body again. Notice the physical sensations, the sounds around you, the thoughts that come and go. Remember to maintain a stance of an observer, without judging or analyzing these experiences.

Step 6: Closing the Meditation
After about 10-20 minutes (or less if you're just starting), prepare to end the meditation. Notice your body and the space around you. Slowly wiggle your fingers and toes, and when you feel ready, open your eyes.

Step 7: Reflect on the Experience
Take a few moments to reflect on the experience. How do you feel physically, emotionally? What was challenging? What did you notice? It might be helpful to jot down your reflections in a journal.

Meditation is a practice, and it's natural to face difficulties. You might struggle with maintaining focus, or you might confront challenging emotions or memories. In these moments, be patient and kind to yourself. With time and consistent practice, mindfulness meditation can become a crucial ally in your journey! Mindfulness forms the backbone of our trauma healing journey. By grounding us in the present, it enables us to break the cycle of rumination that often accompanies trauma. It teaches us to observe our thoughts and feelings without being swept away by them, reducing the grip of past traumas.

Moreover, mindfulness cultivates self-compassion, a crucial ingredient in the recipe for healing. We start to challenge our negative self-talk, treating ourselves with the kindness and understanding we would extend to a loved one. As a result, feelings of guilt or self-blame associated with trauma can be significantly reduced. Mindfulness not only helps us to heal from past traumas but also arms us with resilience to face future challenges. It has proven to be effective in reducing stress and improving mental and physical health - valuable benefits that enhance our quality of life!

Summary:
Mindfulness is the practice of being present and fully engaged in the moment, accepting experiences without judgment. In trauma recovery, it helps anchor us in the present, lessening the power of past events and fears about the future. Mindfulness practices such as breathing exercises, body scans, mindful walking, loving-kindness meditation, mindful journaling, eating, yoga, and guided mindfulness meditation can enhance our awareness, promote self-compassion, and build resilience. Mindfulness is a powerful tool in trauma recovery as it aids in observing our thoughts and emotions without judgment and grounding us in the present moment. This presence helps to interrupt cycles of rumination and enables us to process traumatic experiences healthily. Mindfulness also cultivates self-compassion, challenging negative self-talk and reducing guilt or self-blame, often associated with trauma.

Key takeaways:
1. Mindfulness is the practice of being fully engaged in the present moment, accepting experiences without judgment.
2. Mindfulness plays a crucial role in trauma recovery. It helps anchor us in the 'here and now', breaking the cycle of past and future ruminations, enabling us to process traumatic experiences in a healthy manner.
3. Practices such as breathing exercises, body scans, mindful walking, loving-kindness meditation, mindful journaling, eating, and yoga can help enhance our awareness and ground us in the present.

4. Mindfulness promotes self-compassion, challenging negative self-talk and reducing feelings of guilt or self-blame often associated with trauma.

5. Mindfulness fosters resilience, equipping us with the tools to better handle future challenges.

6. Regular mindfulness practice can reduce stress, a common aftermath of trauma, by promoting a relaxation response.

Chapter 8

Step 7 - Resilience: Building Strength From Struggle

Resilience, simply put, is the ability to bounce back from tough situations. It's not about avoiding struggles; it's about learning to ride the waves and coming out stronger on the other side. As you journey through your trauma healing process, building resilience is like building a muscle, it gets stronger with practicePicture resilience as a life raft, helping you stay afloat during life's storms. When hardships come, as they surely will, resilience allows you to navigate through the storm instead of being drowned by it. Just like a tree bends but doesn't break in the wind, resilient people can sway with life's adversities but remain unbroken. Your experiences, even the most painful ones, are a rich source of strength. Embrace them. Every challenge you've faced and every emotional wound you've endured has made you who you are today. They're not weaknesses but powerful reminders of your strength and ability to overcome. Resilience doesn't mean you won't have moments of despair or vulnerability. On the contrary, acknowledging your feelings and not hiding from them is part of being resilient. It's about getting back up each time you fall, dusting yourself off, and continuing on with even more determination. Finally, remember that resilience isn't a journey you need to undertake alone. Reach out to loved ones, lean on supportive relationships, and don't be afraid to ask for help. The strength to rise from struggle isn't only within you; it's also in the hands of those who care about you. Together, you can build resilience and transform trauma into triumph.

8.1: Understanding Resilience:

Resilience is a term we hear often, but what does it truly mean? At its core, resilience is our human ability to adapt and bounce back when things don't go as planned. It's not about avoiding life's difficulties, but facing them head-on and rising from them stronger and wiser. This chapter is all about understanding resilience and how it plays a crucial role in your trauma healing journey. Imagine resilience as your personal force field, protecting you during life's toughest battles. It doesn't prevent the blows from coming, but it does equip you to handle them more effectively, recover quickly, and continue moving forward. It's akin to being a ship that knows how to sail through the storm, rather than being tossed aimlessly by the waves. Resilience isn't just about surviving; it's about thriving. It's learning how to use adversity as a catalyst for growth and transformation, turning life's stumbling blocks into stepping stones. It's important to understand that resilience is not a trait that people either have or do not have. It involves behaviors, thoughts, and actions that anyone can learn and develop. The ability to become resilient is within us all. To better understand resilience, let's break it down into four key components:

a) Emotional Awareness: Resilience starts with understanding and acknowledging your feelings. It doesn't mean you'll never feel pain, grief, or sadness. It means you allow yourself to feel these emotions and understand that they're a natural part of life's ups and downs.

b) Perseverance: Life is full of obstacles. Resilience involves an unyielding spirit that doesn't give up when things get tough. It's the determination to keep going, no matter how difficult the journey.

c) Self-Care: Resilience requires taking care of your physical and emotional health. This means eating healthily, exercising regularly, getting enough sleep, practicing mindfulness, and doing things that bring joy and relaxation.

d) Supportive Relationships: Building resilience isn't a solo act. Having strong, positive relationships can provide emotional support, lend a different perspective, and help you navigate through challenging times.

Everyone's journey to resilience is different. It's not a linear process but more like a winding road with highs and lows, successes and setbacks. Resilience isn't built in a day; it's built over time. Each step you take, no matter how small, adds another brick to your fortress of resilience. Through resilience, you can learn to channel your inner strength, use your past experiences as a foundation for growth, and forge a path towards healing. It's about taking the raw materials of our experiences - the good and the bad - and creating something beautiful out of them. Remember, resilience isn't about bouncing back to the old you, but bouncing forward to a new, stronger you.

8.2: Strategies for Building Resilience:
Building resilience is a bit like building a house. It requires the right tools, a solid foundation, and time to create something that can withstand life's storms. In this chapter, we'll explore practical strategies to help you construct your resilience 'house', turning trauma into triumph:

a) Embrace Change: Life is ever-changing and sometimes, those changes are challenging. By learning to accept and adapt to changes, we become more flexible and resilient. Remember, change is the only constant, and our ability to navigate through it determines our resilience.

b) Cultivate a Positive Outlook: Try to keep an optimistic attitude, even in tough times. Look for the silver linings and learning opportunities in each experience. A positive mindset helps fuel resilience, allowing us to see beyond our current circumstances and maintain hope for a brighter future.

c) Practice Self-Care: Physical health impacts emotional resilience. Regular exercise, a balanced diet, and adequate rest all contribute to overall wellbeing. But self-care also includes mental and emotional nourishment. Make time for activities you love, practice mindfulness or meditation, and never underestimate the healing power of laughter.

d) Develop Emotional Awareness: Be in tune with your emotions and feelings. Recognize when you're feeling stressed or overwhelmed, and give yourself permission to feel these emotions. Resilience doesn't mean suppressing feelings, but acknowledging them and understanding they're part of the human experience.

e) Nurture Relationships: Strong, positive relationships are a cornerstone of resilience. Don't hesitate to reach out to loved ones for support or offer your support to them. Remember, it's okay to ask for help. Resilience is not about being alone; it's about being connected.

f) Set Realistic Goals: Create achievable goals and take incremental steps towards them. Celebrate each small victory as it comes. The process of setting and achieving goals boosts self-confidence and fosters resilience.

g) Practice Problem-Solving: Develop your problem-solving skills. When faced with a challenge, instead of feeling overwhelmed, brainstorm possible solutions. By focusing on what you can do instead of what you can't, you promote resilience.

h) Cultivate Gratitude: Make it a habit to identify and appreciate the good things in your life, even amidst hardship. Gratitude can shift your focus from what's wrong to what's right, fostering resilience by creating a positive outlook.

i) Seek Professional Help: There's no shame in seeking help from professionals such as therapists or counselors. They can provide valuable tools and techniques to aid your resilience-building journey.

Resilience is not a destination, but a journey. And like any journey, it has its peaks and valleys. But with every step you take, you're becoming stronger and more resilient. You're transforming your struggles into strength, and your wounds into wisdom. Building resilience doesn't mean that you won't experience difficulty or distress. But it does mean that with time, you'll be able to better navigate through the rough seas, recover more quickly, and emerge stronger. Embrace these strategies, be patient with yourself, and remember that you have the inner strength to bounce back better. You are not just a survivor; you're a thriver!

8.3: Case Study: Turning Trauma Into Triumph
The journey of Anna, who turned her trauma into triumph and found resilience within her own story. Her experience serves as a powerful example of how the strategies outlined in this guide can help in healing trauma and building resilience. Anna was a young professional who had faced a series of life-altering traumas. A car accident left her with physical injuries that required extensive therapy and time off work. This incident

was soon followed by the loss of her father. The accumulation of these experiences left Anna feeling overwhelmed, lost, and unable to see past her pain. Despite her adversities, Anna chose not to let her circumstances define her. Instead, she saw them as challenges she had the power to overcome. Her first step in building resilience was accepting her circumstances. She embraced change, acknowledging that her life wouldn't be the same, but it could still be meaningful and fulfilling. Anna actively worked on cultivating a positive outlook. Even on tough days, she practiced finding silver linings. Her physical therapy sessions, for instance, became opportunities to regain strength rather than reminders of her accident. Anna prioritized self-care, recognizing its importance in her healing journey. This included following her physical therapy regimen, maintaining a healthy diet, ensuring she got plenty of rest, and making time for mindfulness exercises and hobbies she loved. She also nurtured her relationships. She leaned on her family and friends for emotional support, and also sought out a support group for individuals who had experienced similar traumas.

Knowing she wasn't alone in her struggle was a significant comfort and provided additional strength. Anna set realistic goals for herself. These included physical recovery targets, like regaining the ability to walk without assistance, and emotional goals, such as allowing herself to grieve her father without guilt. Throughout her journey, Anna continually practiced problem-solving. When she faced a challenge, she took time to brainstorm potential solutions instead of feeling defeated. This proactive approach helped her regain control of her life. Anna also made a daily practice of gratitude. Even in the face of adversity, she sought out things to be grateful for, shifting her focus from what she had lost to what she still had. Finally, Anna wasn't afraid to seek professional help. Regular sessions with a therapist provided her with additional tools to navigate her healing process and continue building resilience. Anna's story is a testament to resilience in the face of trauma. Her journey wasn't without pain, and there were undoubtedly days when it seemed impossible to move forward. But each step she took, however small, added to her resilience and helped her transform her trauma into a story of triumph. Anna's story serves to remind us that we all have the capacity to bounce back better. With perseverance, self-care, emotional awareness, and the right support, it's possible to turn adversity into strength and find resilience amidst our most challenging times.

8.4: Activity: Resilience Reflection Journal:

One of the most powerful tools for building resilience is keeping a reflection journal. Writing allows us to explore our feelings, track our progress, and gain insights about our healing journey. In this chapter, I will guide you to create your own Resilience Reflection Journal.

Starting Your Journal – First, find a notebook that you like. This could be a simple lined notebook or a beautifully designed journal, whichever you feel comfortable with. You can also use digital tools if you prefer typing to writing. It's your journal, and it should reflect you.

Regular Entries – Aim to write in your journal regularly. You don't need to write every day, but try to develop a consistent routine, whether that's a few times a week or every other day. Remember, there's no set amount to write; what matters is that you're taking the time to reflect. What to Write? Here are few examples:

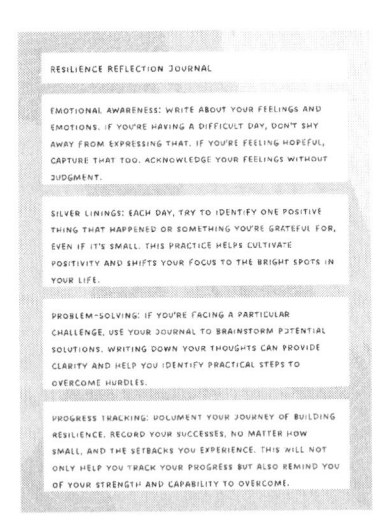

> **RESILIENCE REFLECTION JOURNAL**
>
> EMOTIONAL AWARENESS: WRITE ABOUT YOUR FEELINGS AND EMOTIONS. IF YOU'RE HAVING A DIFFICULT DAY, DON'T SHY AWAY FROM EXPRESSING THAT. IF YOU'RE FEELING HOPEFUL, CAPTURE THAT TOO. ACKNOWLEDGE YOUR FEELINGS WITHOUT JUDGMENT.
>
> SILVER LININGS: EACH DAY, TRY TO IDENTIFY ONE POSITIVE THING THAT HAPPENED OR SOMETHING YOU'RE GRATEFUL FOR, EVEN IF IT'S SMALL. THIS PRACTICE HELPS CULTIVATE POSITIVITY AND SHIFTS YOUR FOCUS TO THE BRIGHT SPOTS IN YOUR LIFE.
>
> PROBLEM-SOLVING: IF YOU'RE FACING A PARTICULAR CHALLENGE, USE YOUR JOURNAL TO BRAINSTORM POTENTIAL SOLUTIONS. WRITING DOWN YOUR THOUGHTS CAN PROVIDE CLARITY AND HELP YOU IDENTIFY PRACTICAL STEPS TO OVERCOME HURDLES.
>
> PROGRESS TRACKING: DOCUMENT YOUR JOURNEY OF BUILDING RESILIENCE. RECORD YOUR SUCCESSES, NO MATTER HOW SMALL, AND THE SETBACKS YOU EXPERIENCE. THIS WILL NOT ONLY HELP YOU TRACK YOUR PROGRESS BUT ALSO REMIND YOU OF YOUR STRENGTH AND CAPABILITY TO OVERCOME.

Emotional Awareness: Write about your feelings and emotions. If you're having a difficult day, don't shy away from expressing that. If you're feeling hopeful, capture that too. Acknowledge your feelings without judgment.

Silver Linings: Each day, try to identify one positive thing that happened or something you're grateful for, even if it's small. This practice helps cultivate positivity and shifts your focus to the bright spots in your life.

Problem-Solving: If you're facing a particular challenge, use your journal to brainstorm potential solutions. Writing down your thoughts can provide clarity and help you identify practical steps to overcome hurdles.

Progress Tracking: Document your journey of building resilience. Record your successes, no matter how small, and the setbacks you experience. This will not only help you track your progress but also remind you of your strength and capability to overcome.

Affirmations: Write down positive affirmations that resonate with you. These could be simple sentences like, "I am strong," "I can handle this," or "I am healing." Reading and writing affirmations can boost your confidence and resilience.

At the end of each week or month, take the time to read your previous entries. Reflect on your feelings, the challenges you've faced, and the progress you've made. What have you learned about yourself? Can you see patterns or insights that might help you moving forward? This Resilience Reflection Journal is your personal space. It's a record of your resilience-building journey and a testament to your inner strength. This journal can help you turn your struggles into stepping stones, paving the way to healing and growth. Resilience isn't a quick process, but rather a journey of small steps leading to bigger leaps. So, even on tough days, know that you're moving forward. With every word you write in your journal, you're taking one more step on your journey. Don't underestimate the power of this tool - it's like a compass, guiding you through the storm towards the light of resilience.

Summary:

"Resilience: Your Trauma Healing Guide" is a comprehensive resource providing practical strategies for overcoming adversity and fostering resilience. By focusing on Emotional Awareness, Perseverance, Self-Care, and Supportive Relationships, the book aims to empower readers to navigate life's challenges effectively and recover quickly. The guide includes the story of Anna, an example of transforming trauma into triumph, and a Resilience Reflection Journal, a tool to facilitate the resilience-building process.

Key Takeaways:
1. Resilience is not about avoiding life's difficulties, but facing them head-on and rising

from them stronger and wiser.

2. Four key components of resilience are Emotional Awareness, Perseverance, Self-Care, and Supportive Relationships.

3. Practical strategies to build resilience include embracing change, cultivating a positive outlook, practicing self-care, developing emotional awareness, nurturing relationships, setting realistic goals, practicing problem-solving, cultivating gratitude, and seeking professional help.

4. Anna's story serves as a powerful example of transforming trauma into triumph through resilience-building strategies.

5. The Resilience Reflection Journal is a helpful tool to facilitate emotional exploration, progress tracking, problem-solving, and positivity cultivation.

6. The journey to resilience is about bouncing forward to a new, stronger self, rather than bouncing back to the old self.

Chapter 9

Step 8 - Growth: Embracing Post-Traumatic Growth

Growth doesn't always come from pleasant experiences; sometimes, it's our struggles that shape us the most. Post-traumatic growth is the silver lining in the storm cloud of trauma. It's the positive psychological change experienced as a result of adversity, leading to a higher level of functioning, personal development, and a deeper appreciation of life. It's not about forgetting or ignoring the pain; it's about acknowledging it and using it as a stepping-stone to become stronger, resilient, and more empathetic. Recognizing this transformative potential is the first step in leveraging it. It requires a shift in perspective: seeing hardship not as a barrier, but as a bridge to a better, stronger version of ourselves. The wounds may leave scars, but they also serve as reminders of our resilience, proof that we've survived, and evidence that we can bounce back.

Embracing post-traumatic growth means finding meaning in suffering, re-evaluating our priorities, strengthening our relationships, and discovering new possibilities. It's about using our pain as a catalyst to propel us into a more enlightened state of being.

Yes, trauma can shatter us, but it also has the potential to rebuild us in ways we could never have imagined. Remember, resilience isn't about how hard you can hit, but how hard you can get hit and still move forward. Growth isn't just about flourishing in good times, but also thriving amidst adversity. In this chapter, we'll guide you in embracing this transformative growth, helping you bounce back better, stronger, and more in tune with your inner strength.

9.1: What is Post-Traumatic Growth?

Simply put, it is the phenomenon of experiencing significant positive change following a traumatic event or a series of challenging life circumstances. PTG isn't about ignoring the pain or hardship you've faced. Rather, it's about embracing the idea that through our most difficult times, we can evolve, grow, and come out on the other side not just intact but stronger and more resilient than we were before. Post-Traumatic Growth is not about returning to your old self, as if the trauma never happened. Instead, it's about bouncing forward, using the experiences and lessons learned to become a newer, stronger, and wiser version of yourself. It's a process of transformation that comes from adversity. However, it's important to note that PTG is not an automatic outcome of trauma. It's not about denying the hurt or hardship that comes with such experiences. Instead, it's about acknowledging these challenges and working through them, not around them. In this transformative journey, individuals often find changes occurring in five primary areas.

First, we see an increase in personal strength. There's a realization that if we can survive the adversity we've faced, we can handle just about anything. This newfound resilience can serve as a powerful tool for facing future challenges. Second, there's often a change in our relationships with others. We might find ourselves feeling more connected to those who have suffered or are suffering. Trauma can heighten our empathy and deepen our connections with others. Third, there's a greater appreciation for life in general. When you've faced significant challenges, you start to appreciate the value of life and the small joys that fill our days. You might find pleasure in things you used to overlook. Fourth, there's the recognition of new possibilities. Trauma can disrupt the path you had set for your life. However, as you recover, you might discover new interests, goals, and pathways that weren't visible to you before. Finally, many experience spiritual growth. This doesn't necessarily mean a religious awakening, but a broader sense of understanding, purpose, or connectedness to the world. In essence, Post-Traumatic Growth is the process of using adversity as a springboard for positive transformation. It's about discovering a new perspective, a fresh appreciation for life, and a deepened sense of strength and resilience. It takes time, patience, and support, but this process can lead to profound personal growth and a life that feels richer, more meaningful, and more rewarding.

9.2: The Process of Post-Traumatic Growth:
PTG isn't about moving on from trauma; it's about moving through it. It's not a magic wand that erases painful memories, but a gradual, intentional process of personal evolution. To begin with, the initial response to a traumatic event is often a period of struggle and distress. You may feel overwhelmed, vulnerable, and uncertain about the future. This is an entirely normal reaction to an abnormal event. Remember, it's okay not to be okay. Allow yourself the space and time to experience your feelings without judgment. The process of PTG often starts when you begin to question and challenge your assumptions about the world and your place in it. This is where the healing journey truly begins. It's about reflecting on your trauma, understanding how it has impacted you, and finding ways to integrate this experience into your life story. Here's how the process often unfolds:

1. Confrontation: You first acknowledge the trauma and allow yourself to experience the feelings associated with it. Confrontation involves recognizing your emotions and accepting that the trauma has changed you. It's about embracing vulnerability.

2. Examination: This is when you begin to question your assumptions about the world, yourself, and others. You start to process what has happened, examine how it has affected your life, and explore the changes in your beliefs and perceptions.

3. Integration: This stage is about finding a way to incorporate the trauma into your life. It involves understanding that the trauma is a part of your story, but it does not define you. You start to see your trauma as a part of your past, something that has shaped you but doesn't constrain your future.

4. Emergence: As you integrate the experience, you begin to see glimmers of growth.

You start to identify changes in yourself, like increased resilience, deeper empathy, and a greater appreciation of life.

5. Flourishing: This is the stage of fully embracing and utilizing your growth. You might find new goals, develop a deeper connection with others, or discover a newfound sense of purpose. It's about thriving in spite of the trauma, using the experience to fuel your personal development.

This process isn't linear, and each person's journey is unique. You may oscillate between stages, and that's okay. What's important is to acknowledge your feelings, be patient with yourself, and seek support when you need it. PTG is about harnessing your adversity and using it as a catalyst for transformation. It's about acknowledging the scars but also recognizing the strength that comes from them. This chapter will guide you through this process, shedding light on the path to a stronger, wiser, and more resilient you. It's about bouncing back better, prepared to face whatever life throws at you with a deeper understanding of your strength and capabilities.

9.3: Tips for Fostering Post-Traumatic Growth:

Embracing post-traumatic growth is not about forgetting or downplaying your pain; it's about using that pain as a catalyst for positive transformation. Here are some tips to help you foster this growth:

1. **Acceptance:** The first step towards post-traumatic growth is accepting that the trauma happened. Denying or minimizing your experiences will only delay healing. Recognize your pain, allow yourself to grieve, and understand that it's okay to not be okay.

2. **Support System:** Surround yourself with people who can provide emotional support. Loved ones, therapists, or support groups can provide a safe space to express your feelings and fears. Sharing your experiences can be cathartic and can help you feel less alone in your journey.

3. **Self-Care:** Physical health and mental health are closely interconnected. Regular exercise, a balanced diet, and plenty of rest can significantly affect your mood and energy levels. Prioritize self-care and treat it as an integral part of your healing process.

4. **Mindfulness:** Practice being present in the moment. Mindfulness exercises, like

meditation or yoga, can help you manage stress, reduce negative emotions, and enhance your emotional resilience.

5. **Journaling:** Writing about your experiences can help you process your emotions and gain perspective. Journaling is a private space where you can express your feelings openly and honestly.

6. **Positive Outlook:** Try to maintain a positive outlook towards life. It doesn't mean ignoring your pain, but focusing on potential opportunities for growth that come with challenges. This perspective can help you remain hopeful and resilient in the face of adversity.

7. **Professional Help:** Don't hesitate to seek professional help. Therapists or counselors trained in trauma can provide you with tools and strategies to cope with your experiences and foster post-traumatic growth.

8. **Patience:** Remember, healing takes time. You don't have to rush through your recovery process. Be patient with yourself and recognize that growth and healing occur at their own pace.

9. **Purpose:** Try to find a sense of purpose in your life. This purpose can help you navigate through challenging times and can provide a sense of direction and motivation.

These tips are designed to guide you on your journey towards post-traumatic growth. They are steps you can take to facilitate your transformation, turning your experiences into a springboard for personal growth and development. Post-traumatic growth isn't about moving on or forgetting about your trauma; it's about moving through it and using it as a catalyst for change. It's about recognizing your strength, building resilience, and transforming adversity into a source of growth.

9.4 Case Study: Real-Life Stories of Post-Traumatic Growth:

We bring the concept of Post-Traumatic Growth (PTG) to life through the experiences of real people. These stories demonstrate the transformative power of PTG, showing that it is possible to not only survive trauma but also to thrive and grow because of it:

Let's begin with the story of Maya. She lost her mother in a car accident when she was just 16. The trauma shook her world, leaving her feeling lost and alone. However, over time, she found a way to channel her pain into a greater purpose. She pursued a degree in psychology, aspiring to help others navigate their grief. The trauma that had once seemed insurmountable had become a catalyst for her personal and professional growth. It's important to remember that Maya's journey was not easy or quick, but her experience demonstrates the power of PTG and the potential for resilience in the face of adversity.

Next, we have the story of Ava, a survivor of a natural disaster. The trauma left her with a heightened appreciation for life and a renewed sense of purpose. She started volunteering for a disaster relief organization, turning her personal tragedy into a source of strength and resilience. Ava's story shows us how trauma can radically shift our perspective, causing us to reevaluate our priorities and find new meaning in our lives.

These case studies underscore the message of this book: that within our darkest moments lie opportunities for remarkable growth. The transformation might not be immediate or easy, but it is possible. With resilience, support, and determination, you can navigate the aftermath of trauma and come out stronger on the other side. You can bounce back better. Remember, you are not alone in this journey. These stories stand as a testament to human strength and resilience, inspiring us to harness our adversities as catalysts for growth.

9.5 Activity: Creating Your Personal Growth Map

We're going to work on a practical and hands-on activity designed to guide you towards post-traumatic growth (PTG). This Personal Growth Map is a visual representation of your journey towards healing and growth. Creating your Personal Growth Map is a powerful tool for self-reflection. It allows you to visualize your path to resilience and recognize the progress you've made. Here's how you can create your own map:

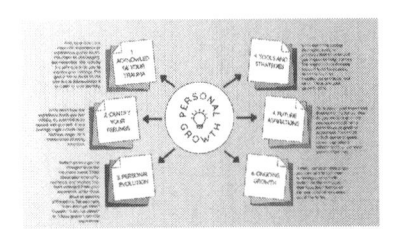

Step 1: Acknowledge Your Trauma
First, note down the traumatic experience or experiences you've faced. This might be challenging, but remember, this activity is a safe space for you to express your feelings. The goal is not to dwell on the pain but to acknowledge it as a part of your journey.

Step 2: Identify Your Feelings
Write down how this experience made you feel initially. It's essential to be honest with yourself. These feelings might include fear, sadness, anger, or a combination of many emotions.

Step 3: Personal Evolution
Reflect on how you've changed since the traumatic event. Think about your strengths, resilience, and wisdom that have emerged from your experience. Write these down as positive affirmations. For example, "I am stronger than I thought," "I am not alone," or "I have grown from this experience.

Step 4: Tools and Strategies
Write down the coping strategies, tools, or practices that have helped you in your healing journey. This might include therapy, support from loved ones, self-care routines, mindfulness practices, and so on. These are your 'growth tools'.

Step 5: Future Aspirations
Think about your hopes and dreams for the future. How do you envision your life moving forward? Write these down as goals or aspirations. This could include personal goals, career aspirations, relationships, or personal growth objectives.

Step 6: Ongoing Growth
Finally, consider what steps you can take to continue nurturing your growth. Reflect on the strategies that have been helpful so far and consider new ones you'd like to try.

Creating this map is an ongoing process. You can keep adding to it as you continue your journey of healing and growth. It's a personal, dynamic document that evolves with you, serving as a visual reminder of your strength, resilience, and capacity for growth. It's a testament to your ability to bounce back better. This activity is not about rushing your healing process or forcing growth. It's about acknowledging your journey, recognizing your growth, and planning for a future shaped by resilience and strength.

Summary:

Emphasizing that the journey of PTG is not linear, the chapter outlines a process of growth, including confrontation, examination, integration, emergence, and flourishing. Tools to foster PTG include acceptance, a supportive network, self-care, mindfulness, journaling, positive outlook, professional help, patience, and purpose. Real-life stories illustrate the transformative power of PTG, showing that trauma can lead to a place of strength, resilience, and new purpose. The chapter ends with an activity to create a Personal Growth Map, a visual representation of one's journey towards healing and growth.

Key Takeaways:
1. Post-Traumatic Growth (PTG) is the process of using adversity as a springboard for positive transformation.
2. PTG involves acknowledging pain and hardship and harnessing them as catalysts for personal evolution and resilience.
3. Changes from PTG can occur in five primary areas: increased personal strength, changed relationships, greater appreciation for life, recognition of new possibilities, and spiritual growth.
4. The process of PTG includes confrontation, examination, integration, emergence, and flourishing.
5. Tools to foster PTG include acceptance, a supportive network, self-care, mindfulness, journaling, maintaining a positive outlook, seeking professional help, exercising patience, and finding purpose.

Chapter 10

Step 9- Maintaining Progress and Preventing Relapse

Maintaining Progress and Preventing Relapse serves as a beacon for your ongoing healing voyage, offering strategies for long-term recovery and relapse prevention. As you navigate life's unpredictable currents, it's crucial to keep hold of the resilience and inner strength you've developed. Challenges might still come, but you're now better equipped to face them without losing your ground. This journey doesn't end at healing; maintaining your emotional balance and well-being is a lifelong commitment. Establishing self-care routines to fortifying your emotional barriers, this chapter guides you on sustaining your healing progress. You'll learn to detect potential pitfalls, respond to emotional triggers healthily, and bounce back if a relapse does occur. The closing chapter of this practical guide reassures you that it's not about never facing adversity again, but about facing it with courage and emerging stronger each time.

10.1: Understanding the Nature of Healing and Relapse:
Healing, at its core, is a process of change and growth. It's about moving from a state of pain and distress towards a state of balance and well-being. As you have walked through the previous eight steps, you've probably already begun experiencing this transforma-

tion. But the key thing to remember is that healing is not linear. There will be days when you feel like you've taken a giant leap forward, and there will be others when you feel like you've stumbled two steps back. And that's okay. It's part of the process, part of the journey. Don't be hard on yourself on the rough days; instead, recognize them as a part of your healing journey and move forward. Relapse, on the other hand, is often viewed with fear and disappointment, which can lead to self-criticism and guilt. It's important to note that experiencing a relapse doesn't mean you've failed or that your efforts have been in vain.

A relapse is not the end of the world; it's simply a reminder that healing is an ongoing process that requires consistent effort and self-care. It's a sign that you need to revisit your healing strategies, perhaps make some adjustments, and reinforce your coping mechanisms. Healing from trauma is like navigating through a labyrinth; there are twists and turns, dead-ends, and U-turns. But each step, each turn, brings you closer to the center - to inner peace and well-being. As such, it's important to view healing and relapse not as opposites, but as complementary parts of the journey. Understanding the true nature of healing and relapse is about accepting the unpredictability of the process and being kind to yourself regardless of where you are in your journey. This understanding will arm you with the right mindset, enabling you to handle the ups and downs with grace and resilience.

10.2: Strategies for Maintaining Progress

The first thing to recognize is that maintaining progress is about consistency. This isn't about monumental leaps and bounds, but rather the small, steady steps that you take every day. It's about showing up for yourself daily and sticking to the practices and strategies that you've found to be helpful in your healing journey. A major strategy is incorporating self-care routines into your everyday life. This could mean taking time each day to meditate, practice mindfulness, exercise, or engage in a hobby that brings you joy. Self-care is not a luxury; it's a necessity. It's about treating yourself with kindness and compassion, replenishing your energy, and creating space for healing. Another crucial strategy involves setting realistic, achievable goals. Setting small, manageable goals gives you a sense of purpose and direction. It provides a roadmap for your healing journey. And each time you achieve a goal, no matter how small, it boosts your confidence and reaffirms your belief in your ability to heal. Building a supportive network is also key. This could be friends, family, support groups, or a trusted therapist. These people can provide emotional support, offer perspective, and remind you of your strength and resilience during challenging times.

Further, it's important to continuously learn and adapt. Stay open to new information, strategies, and techniques that might aid in your healing process. Be willing to adjust your approach as needed, and understand that what works best may change over time. This could involve exploring new therapy approaches, incorporating different mindfulness techniques, or adjusting your self-care routine. Lastly, practice gratitude. It may sound simple, but cultivating a mindset of gratitude can have a profound impact on your healing journey. Regularly acknowledging and appreciating the good in your life can shift your focus away from negative thoughts and emotions and foster a more positive outlook. Maintaining progress in your healing journey is a proactive and ongoing process. It involves nurturing yourself through self-care, setting and achieving goals, building a supportive network, continually learning and adapting, and fostering a mindset of gratitude. Remember, progress may be slow, and there will be inevitable bumps along the way. But with consistency, resilience, and these strategies, you can continue moving forward, ever closer to healing and inner strength.

10.3: Recognizing and Managing Triggers

In the aftermath of trauma, certain situations, environments, or experiences may trigger overwhelming emotions, intrusive thoughts, or physical symptoms reminiscent of your past distress. These are your triggers, and recognizing them is a significant first step in your healing journey. Think of your healing process as walking on a road that you're paving yourself. This road has potholes - your triggers. As you walk, you might sometimes fall into these potholes, causing distress. However, the goal is to identify these potholes, fill them up, or learn to navigate around them. To recognize your triggers, you need to increase your self-awareness. This involves paying close attention to your emotional reactions and physical symptoms. Journaling can be an excellent tool for this, providing a space for reflection and pattern identification.

Once you've recognized your triggers, the next step is managing them. This is not about avoiding or suppressing your triggers, but rather learning to respond to them in a way that minimizes their impact and doesn't derail your healing journey. One key strategy for managing triggers is to practice grounding techniques. These techniques can help you stay present and focused, rather than getting swept up in distressing thoughts or feelings. This could involve deep breathing exercises, mindfulness, or a physical action like touching a piece of jewelry or rubbing your hands together. Another strategy involves cognitive reframing, a technique that helps you change your perspective of the trigger situation. It's about shifting from seeing the trigger as a threat to viewing it as a challenge that you have the strength and resources to handle.

Building a support system is also vital. Having people who understand what you're going through can provide emotional support and reassurance during challenging moments. This could be a therapist, support group, or trusted friend or family member. Remember, managing triggers is not a one-size-fits-all process. It's about finding strategies that work best for you. And with practice, you can get better at handling your triggers, minimizing their impact, and continuing on your healing journey without letting them sidetrack your progress.

10.4: Case Study: Managing Relapse and Coming Out Stronger
Maria, a talented artist, was hit by trauma when her brother tragically passed away. She started therapy and found emotional expression in her art. But healing isn't linear. One day, a picture of her brother triggered a relapse that felt like a tidal wave of grief, seemingly washing away all her progress. Yet, Maria chose to face her pain head-on. She acknowledged her feelings without judgment, remembering it's okay to grieve. She reached out to her support network, leaning on their strength during her time of difficulty. She poured her emotions into her art, a form of catharsis that helped process her feelings. With her therapist, she revisited coping techniques like deep breathing, mindfulness, and yoga. Importantly, Maria reframed her relapse as a part of her healing journey, a chance to deepen her understanding of her trauma, and bolster her resilience. Coming out of the relapse, Maria felt stronger and more self-aware. The experience, while painful, had offered valuable lessons. Healing is a journey; even setbacks can be opportunities for growth. Maria's story embodies the spirit of bouncing back better - through acknowledgment, support, expression, coping strategies, and reframing, we can manage relapse and come out stronger.

10.5: Activity: Developing a Personalized Relapse Prevention Plan

Relapse is a natural part of the healing process, a sign that there's more work to do. It's not a sign of failure, but an opportunity to learn and grow. However, that doesn't mean we can't prepare ourselves to prevent or minimize its impact. This chapter guides you through developing your personalized relapse prevention plan.

PERSONALIZED RELAPSE PREVENTION PLAN

- Identify Your Triggers
- Recognize Your Warning Signs
- Create a Safety Plan
- Build a Support Network
- Practice Self-Care
- Develop Healthy Coping Strategies
- Engage in Therapeutic Activities
- Regularly Review Your Plan
- Remember Self-Compassion

Step 1: Identify Your Triggers: These could be people, places, events, or even certain times of the year that awaken your trauma. Take some time to reflect and list down these triggers. Understanding what these are can help you be better prepared when you encounter them.

Step 2: Recognize Your Warning Signs: Everyone's trauma manifests differently. You might experience certain thoughts, feelings, or physical symptoms that hint at a potential relapse. Knowing these signs can help you take timely action.

Step 3: Create a Safety Plan: Now that you know your triggers and warning signs, create a plan to keep you safe. This could involve removing yourself from a triggering situation, using self-soothing techniques, or reaching out to a trusted friend or family member.

Step 4: Build a Support Network: Healing is easier when you're not alone. Identify people who can support you during difficult times. This could be loved ones, mental health professionals, or support groups.

Step 5: Practice Self-Care: Self-care isn't just about bubble baths and spa days. It's about looking after your physical, emotional, and mental health. This might involve regular exercise, balanced meals, adequate sleep, meditation, or setting boundaries.

Step 6: Develop Healthy Coping Strategies: Find activities that help you relax and manage stress. This could be painting, reading, yoga, mindfulness, or even just a long walk. Use these strategies when you're feeling overwhelmed or notice warning signs of relapse.

Step 7: Engage in Therapeutic Activities: Consider therapies that encourage self-expression and processing emotions, such as art therapy, music therapy, or journaling. These can be useful outlets when you're dealing with intense emotions.

Step 8: Regularly Review Your Plan: Your relapse prevention plan is a living document. As you grow and change, so will your triggers, warning signs, and coping mechanisms. Regularly review and adjust your plan to ensure it still serves your needs.

Step 9: Remember Self-Compassion: Be kind to yourself. Healing is a journey with ups and downs, and it's okay to have difficult days. Remember, each step, no matter how small, is progress.

Creating a personalized relapse prevention plan can give you a sense of control over your healing process. It's a proactive approach that empowers you to take charge of your journey, navigate potential setbacks, and bounce back better. This plan is a testament to your strength, resilience, and commitment to your healing. But remember, it's okay to seek help and lean on others when you need to. You're not alone, and your journey is uniquely yours. No matter where you're at right now, know that each step forward is a step towards recovery. You're doing great, and you're stronger than you think.

Summary:
The guide offers strategies for maintaining progress, such as consistent self-care, setting realistic goals, and building a supportive network. It highlights the importance of recognizing and managing emotional triggers as a key to resilience. A case study illustrates a successful navigation of a relapse, emphasizing the importance of acknowledgment, support, expression, and reframing. The guide concludes with an activity to develop a personalized relapse prevention plan.

Key Takeaways:
1. Healing is non-linear, with both progress and relapse as parts of the journey.

2. Maintaining progress involves self-care, goal-setting, and a supportive network.
3. Recognizing and managing triggers is crucial for resilience and preventing relapse.
4. Relapses can be reframed as opportunities for growth rather than setbacks.
5. A personalized relapse prevention plan can help navigate potential setbacks, providing a roadmap for healing.
6. Regular review and adjustment of the prevention plan ensure its effectiveness over time.
7. Self-compassion and seeking support when needed are integral to the healing journey.

Chapter 11

Moving Forward: Embracing a New Life After Trauma

Recovering from trauma isn't about erasing it, but rather integrating it into your life in a way that allows you to grow and move forward. As you close the pages of this guide, "Bounce Back Better: Your Trauma Healing Guide", it's crucial to remember that your journey doesn't end here. Every day, every step you take is a part of your ongoing journey of healing and growth. You've learned to recognize your triggers, navigate relapses, establish self-care routines, and build a support network. You've developed resilience, learned to face challenges with courage, and discovered your inner strength. Each of these skills and strategies is like a tool in your toolkit, ready to assist you as you embrace your new life after trauma.

As you move forward, remember to treat each day as a new beginning. Understand that it's okay to have tough days, and it's also okay to have joyous days. Both are a part of your journey. Embrace the new chapters of your life, but don't feel pressured to forget the past. It's a part of you, and it's shaped you into the resilient person you are today. Your journey after trauma is a testament to your courage and strength. As you continue on this path, hold onto your hope, nurture your resilience, and believe in your ability to overcome. Life after trauma may look different, but it can be filled with purpose, growth, and happiness. Continue to care for yourself, seek support when needed, and remember, you're stronger than you think. Keep moving forward, for your journey is only just beginning.

11.1: Understanding Your New Normal:

Your "new normal" might look different from what you were accustomed to before experiencing trauma. Perhaps, you're more sensitive to certain triggers, or maybe you've adopted new routines to take care of your mental and emotional health. It might be that you've developed a deeper understanding of your emotions and how to manage them, or you've established a stronger network of supportive individuals around you. Whatever your new normal might look like, it's important to accept it as a valid and crucial part of your journey. The concept of a "new normal" can seem daunting at first. It represents change and the unknown, which can be scary. But it also symbolizes growth, resilience, and the remarkable human ability to adapt. Remember, it's not about comparing your present to your past but about embracing the changes and leveraging them to your advantage.

Recognizing your new normal is the first step. It involves self-reflection and awareness. It requires you to tune into your feelings, observe your reactions, and understand the shifts in your emotional landscape. It can be helpful to maintain a journal, noting down your observations, emotions, and thoughts as you navigate this new phase. Acceptance is the next crucial aspect. Acceptance doesn't mean that you're okay with what happened to you or that you have to forget your past. Instead, it's about acknowledging the impact of the trauma and the changes it has caused in your life. It's about giving yourself permission to move forward, not by leaving your past behind, but by integrating it into your life in a way that allows you to grow.

Adaptation comes hand-in-hand with acceptance. It's about learning to live with your new normal, adjusting your routines, behaviors, and mindset to accommodate the changes. This could mean adopting new self-care practices, engaging in therapy or support groups, or learning new strategies to manage triggers and prevent relapses. Finally, it's about finding joy and purpose within this new normal. While trauma undeniably brings about change, it does not mean that your capacity for happiness, love, and success is diminished. There is room for positive experiences, achievements, and relationships in your new normal. Seek out these positive elements, nurture them, and let them guide you as you forge your path forward.

The journey of understanding your new normal isn't always easy. It requires courage, patience, and perseverance. But remember, this journey is yours, and you're in control. You've already shown incredible strength and resilience by making it this far. As you continue to move forward, keep embracing your new normal, making room for growth, joy, and healing. This new normal doesn't define you, but it does form a part of your story - a story of resilience, healing, and the power to bounce back better.

11.2: Planning for the Future: Goals and Aspirations:
After trauma, setting goals may seem like a daunting task. However, it's important to remember that these goals aren't about returning to your old self or erasing what's happened. Instead, it's about creating a fulfilling future, integrating the experiences and lessons that your trauma has taught you. Start with self-reflection. Ask yourself, "What do I want my life to look like moving forward?" Take some time to visualize your ideal future. It's okay if your vision doesn't come into focus right away. Patience is key. Remember, these aspirations are not fixed; they can change and evolve as you do. Once you have a rough idea, try breaking down this vision into smaller, more manageable goals. These could be anything from developing new hobbies, making career changes, fostering relationships, or adopting healthier habits. The idea is to focus on achievable steps that can bring you closer to your envisioned future.

When setting these goals, ensure they are SMART - Specific, Measurable, Achievable, Relevant, and Time-bound. This helps you to make them concrete, track your progress, and keeps you motivated. For example, instead of saying, "I want to be healthier," you could say, "I will take a 30-minute walk four times a week for the next month." It's essential to remember that goals aren't set in stone. It's okay to adjust them, change them, or even let them go if they no longer serve your needs or align with your journey. Goals are tools to guide you forward, not chains to hold you back. Pursuing your goals will inevitably involve challenges and obstacles. Don't let these deter you. Each challenge is a learning opportunity, and overcoming them is a testament to your strength and resilience. Remember, healing and progress aren't linear. There will be ups and downs, and that's okay. What's important is to keep going, keep trying, and stay committed to your journey.

As you start moving towards your goals, celebrate your achievements, no matter how small. Each step forward, each goal reached, is a victory. These moments of success provide encouragement, boosting your confidence and reinforcing your belief in your capacity to shape your future. Planning for the future also involves practicing self-care and prioritizing your mental and emotional well-being. This might mean continuing therapy, maintaining a support network, and cultivating mindfulness and emotional intelligence. Remember, you're not just planning for a future, you're planning for a healthier, happier you. Lastly, remember to be kind to yourself. Healing is a journey, and it takes time. Don't rush yourself or set unrealistic expectations. Acknowledge your feelings, honor your progress, and be patient with your pace. Setting goals and planning for the future can bring hope and purpose back into your life after trauma. It allows you to take control, to move from surviving to thriving. As you plan for your future, remember your strength, your resilience, and your capacity to bounce back better.

11.3: Giving Back: Helping Others in Their Trauma Journey:
Giving back can be a powerful step in your healing process. It provides a sense of purpose, fosters connection with others, and can reinforce your own learnings and resilience. Seeing your ability to make a positive impact in someone else's life can reaffirm your strength, offering a new perspective on your journey and the value it holds. Start by reflecting on your own experiences and think about what helped you the most. Was it the listening ear of a friend, the wisdom shared by a mentor, or maybe a self-help book like this one that provided practical steps and insights? How can you take these experiences and use them to help others? Consider sharing your story. Opening up about your trauma and your healing journey can inspire others who are facing similar challenges. It lets them know they are not alone, and there is hope. Be mindful, though, to share only when you feel ready and safe, and with those who are receptive and respectful.

You might also provide a supportive presence for those in their healing journey. This could be as simple as being a compassionate listener for someone who needs to talk, or offering to accompany them to therapy sessions or support groups. Remember, it's important not to push someone into sharing if they are not ready. Being supportive means respecting their boundaries and their pace. Additionally, you can involve yourself in community initiatives, support groups, or organizations that help trauma survivors. This can provide a structured way to give back, whether through volunteering your time, sharing your skills, or fundraising for resources.

Giving back doesn't have to be grand or sweeping. Even small acts of kindness and support can make a big difference. The aim is to create a positive ripple, no matter how small it starts. Giving back can also be a process of learning and growth. You may find that in helping others, you deepen your understanding of your own experiences and healing. It's an opportunity to practice empathy, compassion, and resilience. However, while giving back can be fulfilling, it's crucial to maintain your boundaries and ensure you're not neglecting your own needs and wellbeing. Helping others should not come at the cost of your own healing. Listen to your feelings and trust your instincts. If you start to feel overwhelmed, it's okay to step back and focus on self-care. Helping others in their trauma journey is about more than giving back. It's about building connections, growing together, and strengthening your shared resilience. It's a testament to your journey and a beacon for those who are starting theirs. Remember, your story and your strength have the power to inspire, to comfort, and to guide. Through giving back, you can not only transform your own life but also help others to bounce back better from their traumas.

11.4: Activity: Vision Board - Picturing Your Future for Career, Relationships, Travel and Adventure, Health and Wellness, Personal Growth, Hobbies and Passions, Material Possessions.

A Vision Board is a visual representation of your dreams, goals, and aspirations. It serves as a constant reminder of where you want to go and what you want to achieve. Here's how to create one. Start with gathering your materials. You'll need a large piece of poster board or cardboard, a stack of magazines, scissors, and glue. You can also include markers, stickers, or printouts of specific images or quotes from the internet. Take some time to reflect on different areas of your life and what you hope for in each. These areas include:

VISION BOARD

CAREER
What kind of work do you want to do? Do you aspire to climb the corporate ladder?

RELATIONSHIPS
What kind of relationships do you want to cultivate? Think about family, friends.

TRAVEL
Where do you dream of visit? What kind of adventures do you want to experience?

HEALTH
What does a healthy lifestyle look like for you? This can include physical & mental health, etc.

GROWTH
What skills or qualities do you want to develop? This can also include emotional journey.

LIFESTYLE
Are there any specific items you aspire to own? This could be a house, a car, etc.

✳✳✳✳   ✳✳✳✳

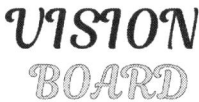

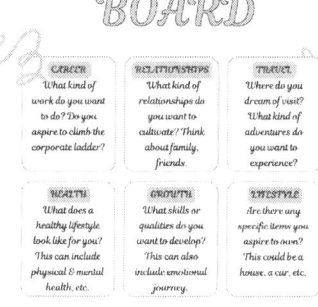

1. **Career:** What kind of work do you want to do? Do you aspire to climb the corporate ladder, launch your own business, or perhaps, make a career change?
2. **Relationships:** What kind of relationships do you want to cultivate? Think about family, friendships, romance, and professional connections.
3. **Travel and Adventure:** Where do you dream of visiting? What kind of adventures do you want to experience?
4. **Health and Wellness:** What does a healthy lifestyle look like for you? This can include physical health, mental health, nutrition, exercise, relaxation, etc.
5. **Personal Growth:** What skills or qualities do you want to develop? This can also include your spiritual or emotional journey.
6. **Hobbies and Passions:** What activities bring you joy and fulfillment? It could be a current hobby or something new you'd like to try.
7. **Material Possessions:** Are there any specific items you aspire to own? This could be a house, a car, or any other material item that symbolizes achievement or success for you.

Once you've reflected on these areas, start cutting out images, words, or phrases from your magazines that represent your goals. Be creative and intuitive in this process. Choose imagery that not only represents your aspirations but also sparks joy and excitement. Arrange your chosen items on your board. There's no right or wrong way to do this. You can group them by categories or mix everything together. The important thing is that the board feels inspiring to you. When you're happy with your layout, start gluing everything down. Now, find a place to hang your Vision Board where you can see it daily. Use it as a source of motivation, a reminder of where you're headed. If you ever feel off track or overwhelmed, look at your Vision Board and remember your bigger picture. Creating a Vision Board is more than just a fun activity. It's a powerful tool for visualizing and manifesting your dreams. It's about recognizing that despite past traumas, you have the power to shape your future. And most importantly, it's a testament to your resilience and ability to be better, stronger, and with a clear vision for the life you desire.

Summary:
Readers are guided through understanding their 'new normal' post-trauma and accepting the changes it brings. They're encouraged to adapt, embrace, and find joy within this new reality, while also learning to set goals and plan for the future. The chapter emphasizes the power of giving back, sharing personal experiences to help others navigate their own trauma journeys. It also introduces the Vision Board activity to help visualize dreams and aspirations across different life areas like career, relationships, health, and personal growth.

Key Takeaways:
1. Understand your 'new normal': Recognize the changes trauma brings and learn to navigate this altered life landscape.
2. Accept and adapt: Accept the impact of trauma and learn to live with your new normal, making adjustments to your routines and behaviors accordingly.
3. Set goals for the future: Envision your future and break down this vision into smaller, manageable goals to create a fulfilling life post-trauma.
4. Give back: Use your experiences to support others navigating their trauma journeys, while maintaining your boundaries and prioritizing your wellbeing.

5. Create a Vision Board: Use this visual tool to represent your dreams and aspirations, reminding you of your goals and serving as a motivation source.

6. Resilience: Despite trauma, you have the strength and resilience to adapt, grow, and shape your future, embodying the ability to 'bounce back better.

Printed in Great Britain
by Amazon